CW00482382

ARMED WITH

Chocolate Frogs

ARMED WITH

Chocolate

Frogs

Living with advanced breast cancer

kate carey
productions

Armed with Chocolate Frogs
ISBN 13: 978 0 9775529 1 7
ISBN 10: 0 9775529 1 8

© copyright in each piece resides with the individual writers, 2006
© copyright in this collection resides with the publisher, 2006

Published by Kate Carey Productions
ABN: 52 579 776 199
51 Ormond Road
Moonee Ponds Vic 3039
Australia
+61 3 9370 6497
katecarey@overthefencepress.com.au
www.overthefencepress.com.au/katecarey

All rights reserved. No part of this publication may be reproduced
without the permission of the publisher.

Creative writing mentor: Christine Gillespie
Publication manager: Tess Moloney
Editor: Debbie Fry
Design by Green Poles Design
Cover image: Jupiterimages
Printed by Everbest

National Library cataloguing-in-publication data:
Armed with chocolate frogs: living with advanced breast cancer.

Includes index.
ISBN 9780977552917 (pbk.).
ISBN 0 9775529 1 8 (pbk.).

1. Breast - Cancer - Australia. 2. Cancer - Patients
- Australia - Biography. 3. Breast cancer patients' writings
- Literary collections. I. Title.

305.4092

DEDICATION

*To those who live with breast cancer, to those who died from it,
and to their families and friends who support them.*

*For Noni, Sue, Joanna, Carol, Liz, Angela –
we could fill a page and more.*

Foreword

Armed with Chocolate Frogs is a powerful and moving collection of writing from women across Australia whose breast cancer has travelled to other parts of their bodies.

In 2003, Breast Cancer Network Australia funded two Inspirational Women with Advanced Breast Cancer writing workshops. By teleconference and email, twenty women from around Australia worked with professional writer Christine Gillespie to write from the heart about some of their experiences of living with cancer.

The personal journeys of the women who contributed to this collection are presented in vignettes and poetry. Collectively they provide powerful insights into the daily battles faced by women living with secondary (metastatic or stage four) breast cancer. The writers wanted to share their stories with others. They know that there are thousands of women around Australia living with secondary breast cancer. Many women live for years with this often chronic and progressive illness. Many feel very alone in their journey. Few support groups exist and there are few resources. If you are living with secondary breast cancer, or are a family member or friend of someone who is, we hope *Armed with Chocolate Frogs* is a source of connection, support and inspiration. We also hope it assists health professionals to gain further insight into the sorrows and the joys of those living with secondary cancer.

Those who participated found the workshops invaluable: there were challenges and rewards, tears and laughter, pain and catharsis. The workshops not only produced this fine collection, they also led to other positive outcomes for the women who participated. They learned to write creatively, and many have continued to use these skills beyond the workshops. They learned that in the process of writing about their journey with breast cancer, many previously unexamined experiences could be explored and documented. Some women shared their work with family members, which then led to conversations that helped to foster a shared understanding of the emotional journey they were on as a family. For some women this was the first opportunity they had had to talk with other women who shared a similar diagnosis and some strong friendships were formed.

As the project manager, it was an incredible privilege to work with, and come to know, many of the women who participated in the writing workshops. I have admired their courage and determination to live life to the full despite the ongoing intrusions of their illness. I have also marvelled at their determination to make a difference for others who are living with secondary breast cancer. It is a testament to their determination that this book has been published.

Whether you are a woman living with secondary breast cancer, a family member, friend, or a health professional, I am sure you will find this book to be a source of inspiration.

MARY HARVEY

Contents

Veronica Macaulay-Cross

Probably nothing

I remember the moment I discovered the lump in my breast. I was at Phil's unit for a long weekend. He lived in Sydney, and I in Brisbane. We were commuting regularly to spend time with each other, enjoying our romance. In hindsight, it was just as well I was at his place. It was his bathroom mirror, you see. It was large and modern, well lit, with those fancy lights you see in film stars' dressing rooms. Sitting just above the vanity basin, you could see yourself from the waist up. Whereas my mirror at home was small and old-fashioned, in front of a white medicine cabinet. All you could see was your face. There I was, bending over the vanity, brushing my teeth. Dressed in only my underwear, I looked up and noticed a raised lump sitting high in my left breast, above the bra. I stopped brushing and looked across at my right breast. Nothing like it on that side. My fingers felt the lump. It felt like a bubble – not hard, but soft and fluid.

I showed the bubble to Phil. He could feel and see it too. We were certain it was nothing to worry about – just a cyst or something. But, we agreed I should see my GP as soon as I got home.

A few days later, Phil rang and asked if I'd been to the GP yet. I said no, as I'd been too busy with teaching and looking after my ten-year-old daughter. He insisted I go.

My GP is about my age – forty at that time, and his son is the same age as my daughter. He had heard about my marriage breakdown. Bad news always travels fast! I excitedly told him of the new man in my life. He looked at the lump and examined me. It was probably nothing, but to be on the safe side he'd send me for a mammogram. My first mammogram.

I had to leave school for a few hours in the morning. It was the only appointment I could get. At the clinic I was asked to change into a gown (green or pink) and then wait in a room with tables and chairs with about twenty other women, all in coloured gowns, drinking coffee and reading magazines. A volunteer came and asked me if I'd like a tea or coffee.

I had my mammogram and waited. I had an ultrasound. Then I waited again. The waiting room started to empty. I got anxious. The volunteer chatted to distract me. Why did they want me to stay, when most other people had left? Eventually, a doctor came and told me to stay and see the specialist. I was really worried now.

The specialist had my mammogram x-ray up on the light board. He told me there were two suspicious areas in the left breast and they were almost certain it was breast cancer. He asked me if there was any family history. None I was aware of. He advised me to see my GP for a referral to a breast surgeon as soon as possible.

I drove back to work, stunned. At school, it was difficult to act as if there was nothing wrong. I confided in my good friend and told the head of department. I packed my briefcase and off-loaded some marking onto my colleagues. Little did I know then I would not return to work for six months.

A few weeks later, after the mastectomy and the commencement of chemotherapy, one of my colleagues visited me at home. He had a beautiful bunch of flowers and a card. He kept asking me to open the card, but I said I'd open it later, as I thought I might cry reading their messages. Later, when he'd gone, I opened the card. I was absolutely flabbergasted to find over $1,000 cash!

My colleagues (there were over one hundred and fifty teachers at the school) had taken up a collection to buy a present for me. They told me people just kept coming up and giving them money, so they decided to give me the cash instead. It certainly amazed and touched me. It is one of those moments which stays with me always.

Up and away

For the first time in seven days, I woke up feeling better. I lay quietly in my hospital bed, looking out the window at the early, hazy morning. My mind was still and I felt peaceful.

Suddenly a big, bright, orange hot air balloon filled the square and gently floated across the inner city skyline. I sat up quickly, got out of bed and walked to the window. How easy it was. My back was not aching and I could actually stand up without bending over to accommodate my hip-to-hip stitches. Watching the balloon, I longed to be in the basket, gently floating and flying up, up and away. At that moment, I knew I could overcome my troubles – a radical modified mastectomy of my left breast and a tram flap reconstruction★.

For a few seconds, I was part of the beautiful balloon, living in the moment.

★   In a tram flap reconstruction, skin, fat and muscle is taken from the lower half of the abdomen to reconstruct a breast.

Bittersweet

We slept in the back room on my first night home from hospital. It has more light and a better view of our fifties-style backyard. No designer landscaping for us! Umbrella, red hibiscus, yellow cassias, tall palms, green grass, the old Hills hoist and the fragrant herb bed with its rosemary and lavender. At the end of the narrow yard, just in view, were old gums, mangroves and a tidal creek. The moon was full and on the rise – a bright, mellow, golden orb. A black flying fox swooped low into the umbrella blossoms and I heard the flap of wings. Then, it was quiet. Bittersweet being home!

Phil was fussing, tense and worried. He was usually relaxed. Gently he helped me into our inviting bed and I reached out my arms for him to join me. We embraced and kissed, together again. I felt safe and loved, but full, wet tears forced their way out of my eyes. I sobbed for my lost breast and good health. Phil gently wiped my eyes and held me tight. His voice was soothing, his grey-blue eyes loving.

'I love you and we are in this together. I don't love you any less because you have lost a breast. Nothing has changed between us. We will fight this together.'

Gradually I relaxed, and slowly drifted into a relieved and peaceful sleep.

A bit of a problem

The waiting room of the Haematology and Oncology Clinic was nearly empty. It was painted in calming green with purple trim, which could not disguise the lurking treatment rooms. My appointment was for four o'clock but it was now half past five. I was done with reading the tired women's magazines and I'd telephoned Phil to tell him of the delay. The pictures on the wall were nondescript. Splashes of colour, abstract, extravagantly framed. I couldn't relate to them. Most of the receptionists were leaving – a spring returning to their step. After three years of review, I'd almost learnt to curb my impatience. Finally my oncologist appeared.

'Veronica, come in. How are you feeling? Any more pain in the hip?'

'No,' I said, 'It's gone.'

After I was seated, he said, 'We've got a bit of a problem here.' He looked tired and for the first time, I noticed that his hair was very grey. He had aged a lot in the three years I'd been visiting. I waited for him to finish, still not particularly worried.

He continued, 'The scans show that you have metastatic breast cancer in your lumbar spine.'

I was amazed. I felt like I was in a nightmare. It was almost like an out-of-body experience. I looked at his serious face and fought back tears.

'You call that a bit of a problem!' It was hard to joke.

My second marriage

he first time I married, I was twenty-one. Young, with the world at my feet. I was rebellious and married in a registry office, with my husband's sisters and their boyfriends for witnesses. I wore a shiny white blouse, dark velvet slacks and a grey, pinstripe blazer. My bouquet brimmed with tuberoses, little white carnations and white ribbons. I sometimes look at the old photos. A young woman, with long blond hair and a beautiful, innocent face. My ex with his wavy shoulder-length hair. When our daughter was little, she'd point at the photo and say, 'That's Daddy when he was a little girl!'

Twenty-two years on and I was getting married again. Still a simple wedding, but in a church this time, with all my relatives and friends. I had planned to wear an understated, pink, light wool suit, but by the time we'd organised the wedding, it was October and warming up. I stressed about what to wear, but had little energy to shop or fuss, as I was on second-line chemotherapy. On the Wednesday before the wedding, my mother arrived and said, 'Come on. Get ready. I'm taking you shopping to my boutique. They always have some wonderful things there!'

I thought, 'Oh great! A boutique for matrons. Just what I need. I'll end up looking like a frump!'

The sales assistant was an older blond woman, and very helpful. I told her I had to attend a fairly formal wedding on Saturday and had nothing to wear. I glared at my mother with the unspoken message not to tell her it was my wedding. The sales assistant looked me up and down. She returned with a pale, mushroom pink, three-piece outfit. A long skirt in two layers of filmy, floating material – very flattering. An under-top and a beautiful, long sleeved over jacket with simple embroidery, all made of the same soft fabric. I thought it looked okay and quickly decided to take it. I was tired and worried I'd lose my wig, trying things on.

My mother said, 'Are you sure? You've only tried on one outfit!'

On the morning of the wedding, my husband-to-be was working with friends in one of their kitchens, peeling prawns, cooking finger food, delivering things to the hall. Another friend had stayed up all night arranging flowers for the church and hall. She wanted them to be fresh.

I got dressed in my pale pink outfit. Then I secured my blond, bob wig and put on my new pearl jewellery. The outfit was perfect. But my wig looked plain. I tore down the front stairs and picked a small, white gardenia, fresh from the garden and placed it above my right ear.

In the mirror I could see that young innocent woman looking out at me! She is there in the wedding photos too, along with her bridesmaid daughter, her parents, his parents, and their wonderful relatives and friends.

Freedom

*W*e wait on the pontoon at the mouth of the creek. I hear a noise and look up. There, on the top of the narrow jetty post perches a pelican, his soft pink eyes surveying the scene. I laugh and motion for Phil to look.

The tide is in and the sun is glittering on the rippling water. Phil shades his eyes with his hand, watching. Ken manoeuvres our new white boat alongside. We leap into action, fending the boat off while Phil jumps aboard, smiling and eager. I take my time. Both men reach out their arms to help me carefully aboard.

Ken pushes the throttle forward and the motor drones. We're off through the heads, heading for the bay. Phil laughs and talks loudly. He is so excited. I hold on tight as the boat gets up speed and bangs on the small waves. Ken shouts over the noise and motions for Phil to look as he sets a course on the GPS.

My mind wanders to my past yachting days when I was fit and trim and strong. I could anchor, keep my footing on a heaving deck, haul on halyards, take the tiller in club races and cook the grub below. We sailed to some magical places. The freedom of boating.

We hold on tight as Ken puts the boat through its paces. He is sad to be selling, but Phil has assured him he always has a berth on board. An extra pair of hands will be necessary. I sit up straight in the seat, square my shoulders and promise myself that I will be extra careful.

Once again my mind wanders. I can see Phil, my daughter, her boyfriend and myself on our boat. We anchor in clear blue water over clean yellow sand. We gear up to go snorkelling on the old, jagged, rusty wrecks. The sand hills and the bush of the island stand tall, reaching down to the beach where the water gently laps. The sun is shining and reflects off a fishing rod, standing at the ready…

Before BC

*Y*ou're a loser,' yells my sixteen-year-old daughter. 'Just shut up!'

I feel the knife twist and turn in my heart, which shelters behind my reconstructed breast. (This breast sits up, firm but nippleless, while the other droops, soft and warm.)

'How can you say that to me, after all I have been through?' I yell through her closed door.

'Oh, you've been talking about dying for six years!' she shouts.

'I have not and you know it. I've been talking about living! It is only three years since my metastatic diagnosis. I can't help it if the doctor says there is no cure. I'm doing quite well. Anyway, this is about your homework and jobs, not my breast cancer!'

I wonder what our neighbour thinks. My daughter's bedroom is just near her house. I sigh. The loud music, the shouting! She must be used to it by now!

'Oh, go away, I want to sleep!'

I plod up the stairs. I feel so desperate. I want these years with my daughter to be happy and loving. I want my daughter to seize the day with me. But I also want her to learn to accept responsibility, do things for herself and contribute to the household chores. Where did I go wrong? She doesn't seem to respect me; she seems to hate me. Someone, maybe the psychologist, said that she might be pushing me away because she can't bear to lose me. It doesn't feel like that to me. Doesn't she realise how difficult it is for me? The relentless monthly treatments, the needles in uncooperative veins, the six-monthly scans which set me on edge for a week before, the medication, the fatigue, the weight gain, the sore hands and feet! Doesn't she see how well I am coping, making the best of things, striving to live joyfully, being there for her, supporting her in her final school years?

For six years my breast cancer has been intruding on her life. She says she just wants to be normal like the other girls and have a mother without breast cancer. I say, 'What is normal? This is normal!'

She is prone to being a drama queen! Yet, I realise she probably hardly remembers me before BC. I remember her. She was chubby and laughing, always singing! Her eyes lit up and her shiny cheeks dimpled as she recounted a story from the school day. Her teacher, Mrs Jenkins, called her 'a notice box'! But my daughter didn't mind. She laughed. Her favourite food was spaghetti bolognaise. She loved swimming and the beach, her little belly protruding from her two-piece suit. She loved her friends and played games. She knew her favourite videos off by heart. She listened to me and believed what I said. She loved me and I could see the devotion in her eyes.

'Don't fret,' my friends and family say, 'She will grow up and one day, when she is twenty-two or so, you'll be great friends!'

Another six years away! I pray to God I live another six years!

Mary McGregor

Chocolate frogs

Fear

'Celebrate the anniversaries,' they told me.

There was nothing to celebrate twelve months ago. What a sick, sinking feeling it was when the word cancer was shoved in my face.

This was not in my plans. I had a trillion things to do in my life. I wanted to work until I didn't want to do it anymore. I wanted to travel and see all those exotic places I had not yet visited. I wanted to have extended time on my remote island getaway. I wanted…I wanted…

The Expensive Champagne Club has taken every opportunity to celebrate over the last months. Champers and support were essential ingredients for my recovery, but they did not dissolve the deep-seated fear that took over my whole being. Fear that made my head spin, my heart pound, my body ache, my brain scramble, my emotions fragile.

I can say to myself over and over:

Stop this stupid nonsense. Get over it. Stop jabbing yourself with fear. But the fear never goes away. I feel like a hypochondriac.

I won't tell anyone. My friends must be sick of my complaints.

Every ache and pain, no matter how minor, becomes monumental. Is my body at it again? What is it doing now? What is that soreness in my legs, my back, my wrists? Everywhere. The imagination goes wild.

They say that it is harder to cope post-treatment. How true. I am desperate to leave during treatment, but without the day-by-day, week-by-week support there is plenty to dwell on when I'm alone.

I must stay positive and convince myself that everything is fine, even when I can feel my body falling apart. Self-talk works. I know that. I wonder whether the fear will diminish with time. I hope so.

In the meantime, I will celebrate the anniversaries. There must be one coming up soon. I must check.

Hair raising

*W*hat!…Bald? I have just spent $150 on a colour and cut and you are telling me that I am going to lose it all in a month?

The first offering from my friends was an old Davy Crockett hat. We laughed and demonstrated how it could be worn. Then I tried shopping for a wig; that was no fun. They all looked like possums on my head. They itched, caused hot flushes – also known as power surges – and were unstable in high winds. It was a bad mistake to shop for a wig on my own. It was hard to keep hold of the emotions. I cried a torrent of tears at my friend's door afterwards.

The second attempt with two friends was more successful. I even wore the wig home on top of what was left of my fragile hair. Nobody stared at me. How come? Did no one realise that I had a wig on? Possibly not! Everyone had to try the wig, but it looked better on me than on my friends. The belly laughs were therapeutic.

By now hair was coming out in clumps. Thank God I did not have my waist-length hair to cope with or I would probably have been strangled by it in the middle of the night. Ugly, ugly, ugly. Bald patches where my hair used to be. Didn't have to spend $150 at the hairdresser this time. The number eight crew cut on the top and the number four at the back were free. How strange it felt. I was brave enough to be hairless in public where I was not known, but the wig was essential at work and at social events.

Soon, the crew cut looked patchy. I needed a shave. The hairdresser came to my place. There was very little left to fall on the kitchen floor, but the bit that did was to be my last hair for many months. I had never been a fan of bald men, and now I had become a bald woman. I often wondered whether bald men polished their heads. I now think not.

Months later my head was covered with very fine white hair. Where did this come from? I had not totally finished chemotherapy, but had gone onto a different variety. I knew I was going grey, but this whiteness was too much!

The white slowly turned to dark roots, to black speckled with grey, and curls! Now come on! I had spent at least thirty years of my life with waist-length dead-straight hair. My mum had straight, fine, mousy brown hair. My dad had coarse black curls. It was amazing. My hair had changed from my mum's to my dad's. How could this happen?

I have hair back now and I do not have to wear the possum anymore. Maybe one day, my hair texture might go back to what it was. If it doesn't, I don't care. I have saved a bucket of money on hairdresser's appointments over the last twelve months. I have not gone grey gracefully. There is no grace in chemo greying. But now I don't feel that I have to colour my hair. It is amazing what positives can come out of the negatives.

The profession

From my bed I looked up at my surgeon with disbelief and defiance. Couldn't he admit that I was in hospital because of an infection from surgery? My medical knowledge is limited, but I knew how awful I had felt over the last five days. 'What else could be the cause?' I asked. No answer.

A decade-and-a-half ago, I had post-surgery complications with a knee reconstruction. What is it with professionals in the surgical field who can't admit that this stuff happens?

I do have the highest respect for those in the medical profession. In the last year-and-a-half my general practitioner, breast surgeon and oncologist have saved my life. Years ago my orthopaedic surgeon allowed me to continue to play competitive sport long past my scheduled retirement date. However, it's fascinating that the professionals can't see that a surgical problem might relate to the surgical procedure. I have spoken to many people who have said they have experienced similar situations.

I just want an answer

I can't wait two more days. I screamed hysterically over and over again, 'It's not fair. It's not fair.' Part of me wondered whether next door or those in the street could hear. My breast surgeon had just cancelled today's appointment and rescheduled for Thursday. The results of last Friday's tests were incomplete. My heart raced and my stomach churned thinking of another forty-eight hours of uncertainty. Hunched up in my lounge room I raged. For the last six days I had held it together, but right now, all my strength and bravado crashed down around me. I also had the guilts. I had been less than polite to my breast surgeon on the phone.

'You will have to wait,' he said.

'I just want to fucking *know*. Why can't you tell me?' I shrieked through the tears and panic. 'If I do have breast cancer I want treatment. Starting now. If I don't have breast cancer then let's sort out what's wrong,' I yelled. 'So I can get on with my life.'

I was in limbo. My mind was racing ahead, adjusting my life. Can I continue at work? Can I keep playing sport? Will I be alive at Christmas and, more to the point, why me? I rang my GP and poured out my frustrations. It felt good to do *something*! My breast surgeon rang again within fifteen minutes to say that he would meet with me late tomorrow, but with no promises of an answer. I apologised for my uncouth behaviour.

Within twenty-four hours, the diagnosis was confirmed as inflammatory breast cancer. 'Okay, let's go!' I said. I was calm as I listened to the proposed treatment. Calm turned to panic and a scrambled mind. Nine months. Nine months' treatment. There was still a second full day of tests to go. Blood tests and CT and bone scans provided the first good news – the cancer had not spread. I celebrated stage three (not stage four) breast cancer. My friends and I drank the best bottle of champagne we could find and I was on the road to recovery.

Annie Hall

Chocolate frogs

MRI madness

I lie on the bed as it moves in
to scan my spine, my neck, my brain.
Jackhammers, up close and personal,
shake my whole body.
My heart is about to stop.
No music. Can't hear the music.
Don't panic. Try not to panic.
I count the thuds.
Five hundred and still going.
Six hundred, eight hundred,
one thousand.

Please God let me be okay.
I still have songs to sing,
people to help,
lavender to plant.
The jackhammer stops.
The technician says 'Oh sorry,
I forgot to turn up the music.
Why didn't you tell me?'
'Never mind, it's not important,'
I say.

What a support

When I attended my first support group in 1996, I couldn't get through my first sentence without the tears falling. I was very frightened, having been diagnosed with early breast cancer. The women were friendly. I continued going until I felt that I had told my story often enough. I wanted to be able to chat more informally.

I now attend a monthly support group for advanced breast cancer, an hour's drive away. The time passes quickly as I chat with my two friends in the peak hour traffic.

We arrive at the 'chemo cottage', a glorious old house with high ceilings and leadlight windows. Pat, our friendly, caring facilitator, greets us at the door and asks how our journey was after coming 'all that way'! Pat had early breast cancer many years ago, so she has been along part of our path. We have juice, wine, tea, coffee, or water, and perfect little sandwiches to nibble on. It's like a friend's lounge room as we sink into the comfy chairs. Pat guides the group, making sure that one of our golden rules is adhered to; one person only to speak at a time.

Our first evening was labelled 'art therapy'. We felt like school children as we were given butchers' paper and crayons in every colour. I couldn't comprehend what it was all supposed to mean, but I dutifully drew my little stick figures!

We had 'Christmas in July', a wondrous evening where the nurses and Pat cooked a turkey, with crisp baked potatoes, mouth-watering vegetables, plum pudding with custard, yummy nibbles, silver cutlery and shiny wine glasses. They did this for us. We pulled bonbons, put hats on our heads and read silly jokes out loud. Then we clinked glasses and drank to each other's health.

On our support evenings, there's a look, a nod of the head – someone else has been there also. We speak freely.

The evening ends and Pat gives us airline cups of apple juice and wraps a few sandwiches in serviettes, 'for the journey home'. Some ladies ask us if we are staying the night in Sydney…but we are brave and head off up the mountain!

Nice to see you again!

The oncologist kept putting the edge of her hand on the desk, measuring distance on its surface. 'Statistically, your life will end here,' she stated, slicing with her hand, as though she was describing the life of a light globe or a pair of shoes.

My mind blurred. I got up.

'It was nice to see you again.' I left the office.

Innate politeness. Untrue words. So untrue.

I needed sunshine. Sunshine and air. The breeze on my face to assure me that I was still a part of this world.

'I feel so terrible after that.'

'Because she was talking about death?' My sister guided me to a seat in the garden. Alongside me, the beds were covered with thousands of cigarette butts.

'No. She kept talking about my date of death as though she knew when that would be.'

'Well, everyone has to die sometime.'

'Yes, but she doesn't know when that will be for me, anymore than I know when it will be for her. Why is she playing God?'

Heart and soul

He leaned back in his chair, hands behind his head. Twenty-one days after diagnosis of metastatic breast cancer, I was in the oncologist's office struggling to fathom what he was saying. All that was needed to complete the picture was for him to put his feet on the table.

'I wanted to ask about neck massage,' I said.

'Yes, as long as they don't dig into your neck and break it.'

The shock must have shown on my face because his next words were, 'Well, you did ask my opinion.'

He asked me how I felt.

'Quite happy,' I said.

'But you're ringing here every five minutes.' He spat the words out.

'I beg your pardon,' I spluttered. 'I have rung three times in three weeks, two of those times to get results. I didn't expect such rudeness from you!'

Time stood still. My brain was in a fog. What do I say? What do I do? There is no one else to hear this. Would he have said those words if my husband or a friend had been with me? I wished I had a small tape recorder tucked under my shirt.

He continued, 'In a few months' time, you should only be thinking about cancer the day before you come for a visit.'

What...planet are you on, you moron, my brain screamed. The words didn't come out. Again my politeness. I am too bloody polite.

I thanked him. *Thanked him!!!* Do you believe it?

I walked out, every cell protesting, quivering in rage, until I reached my car. I punched the numbers into my mobile to reach my husband. Could barely speak, hardly get the words out.

My saviour of the moment, my dear friend Marg, walked past. She enveloped me in a hug and took me for a coffee. The hot liquid and the talking calmed me down eventually, soothing my soul, and restoring my shattered heart.

Leona Furstenburg

Knowing my body

I have checked my breasts on a regular basis since I was twenty-seven, not only to learn about my body, but also to be able to detect any changes as early as possible. My GP had suggested I participate in the hospital's screening program because of my family history with not only breast cancer, but ovarian cancer too. Since my mother died from breast cancer in 1987 at fifty-one, my awareness of breast cancer had dramatically increased. But as it turned out, obviously I had not been as thorough as I should have.

Six years later, I had changed jobs, moved from outback Queensland to Brisbane, and life was stressful. I had not been feeling well so I went to my doctor several times over a couple of months. All tests came back normal. On one of my trips to her, I was walking up the hill and I thought, what if I had breast cancer? I quickly put it out of my mind; don't be silly, I said, I'm too young! Little did I know!

I had felt a change to a previously diagnosed fibroid adenoma in my right breast. My doctor didn't feel any change, but she examined me thoroughly. 'What's this?' she said. She had found a large lump high in my armpit. Good thing I was lying down. I had always checked my breasts, but had not felt in the armpit area.

The next day, I was at the hospital for an ultrasound and mammogram. I didn't need these tests to tell me I had breast cancer. I just knew.

The following day I sat in the retreat, a sunny bright room with a large comfy couch, awaiting the consulting doctor and a verdict that would not go my way.

Two years and two months later, at thirty-four, my worst nightmare was realised. I had been for my six-monthly check-up and everything was clear. Ten days later I went for a remedial massage. The massage therapist I had been seeing for almost two years quietly said to me, 'What's this lump on your neck?'

'Don't use that word lump, I have an aversion to it!' I said.

I went to my local GP. She knew my medical history but suggested waiting eight weeks to see what would happen to the lump. She thought it might be a reactive lymph node since I'd had a tooth pulled just days before, slightly infected and on the same side. I was uneasy with the advice. I waited a tense three weeks and then asked my husband to come back to the GP with me for moral support in case she would not go further with testing. However, she suggested an ultrasound.

I lay on the bed, the room darkened so the technician could see the screen as she went over the area. Not only was there the lump that I could feel, but also two other lumps swollen underneath. I knew in my heart the disease had returned. A day later it was confirmed.

A woman should know her body and go with her instincts; she has to ensure that doctors listen to her. Breast cancer is such an insidious disease; it takes instinct and courage to detect it and fight it. Know your body!

It comes in threes!

*I*t was 8 February, 2000. A normal Tuesday evening. We had just finished dinner and were sitting down to watch television when the phone rang. 'It's probably for you,' my husband said. It usually is!

This time it was for him. It was his mother telling us she had been diagnosed with bowel cancer. Mum was in her sixties and had fought her way through breast cancer in 1994. We knew it would be hard on her, but she would get through it. This was the same day I had been to the breast clinic. I would get my test results the next day. My husband, Roy, had flown up from Canberra where he was working to be with me. No one else knew about the tests.

The following morning at seven, I went with my father to his doctor to get the results of some tests he had taken earlier that week. I left Roy in the garden attending to the roses. I guess it was giving him something to do while he waited for me to return home. It was a cheerful kind of Queensland day, the sun shining brightly, the birds chirping away in the trees.

Dad's results were not good. We sat in two large stuffy chairs facing the doctor. He gave us the news in a matter-of-fact sort of way. Dad had prostate cancer. We left the doctor's room with our arms around each other. I was trying to give Dad the comfort I knew he needed, but I didn't know if it was helping him. Life is tough at times. We said our goodbyes outside. I sat in the car and cried.

I went home to pick up Roy, who was now showered and dressed, ready to go to my nine o'clock appointment. So far things were not going well.

On that morning I was told I had breast cancer. My husband was by my side. I knew I had a battle on my hands. Through my tears I remember the doctor telling me that things were different now from when my mother was ill. Treatments had changed; progress had been made in the world of breast cancer.

Why three diagnoses in less than twenty-four hours? I will

never understand. This can be a cruel world. The next challenge was to tell each of our families what had happened.

I could not tell my father. I found it too difficult to tell him, on the day he was told he had prostate cancer, that his only daughter had breast cancer, thirteen years after his wife had died from the disease.

Telling Roy's daughter with whom I share a loving and caring relationship was very hard. She was shocked to see me walk in the door with Roy, knowing that there must have been a reason for him to be home from Canberra in the middle of the week. Her first reaction was that her grandmother had died. No, she had bowel cancer and I had breast cancer.

We are all dealt certain cards in life, from where I will never know. The challenge is there and I take it up. I have too much to live for and I am certainly not about to give up!

Crying alone

I lay on the bed, curled up after the eighth of twenty-two radiotherapy treatments. My skin was sensitive to touch, crawling and irritating. Tears flowed down my face and onto my burning chest. My arm was hurting. I knew all this would happen before I started treatment. I had done it all three years ago. Why was it happening again?

The door to my bedroom opened gently. Max, my eighteen-month-old golden retriever, snuck into the room. He approached me tentatively. Being in here was not allowed, but this time was an exception. He placed two paws on the bed, looking at me with his big brown eyes. Why was I crying?

I cried and cried. I needed to let those tears out; I needed that release. Max climbed onto the bed, drew close and lay next to me. He licked my left hand once, and then started licking my right hand, the side that was being attacked by breast cancer for the second time. He was such a comfort to me that I let it all out. Afterwards, I felt better. I felt stronger.

I can fight this. I can beat this. I am a young woman, and with Max by my side, I can get through it.

My friends

My friends – what would I do without them? The phone rings, what are you doing on Friday? Let me check my diary! No I'm serious, I can't remember what's on that day. Doctors' appointments, huh! Lunch, coffee, shopping, movies. Now you're talking! They ring to say hello. They ring to say they care.

My friends are special. My friends are unique. My friends, above all else, love me as I am, care for me as I am, and will always be there for me.

And so to my many friends, I say, thank you with all my love.

That day

I was in love, I was happy!

I was working part-time as a receptionist for a small inner city firm with a staff of about twelve people. I enjoyed the job; it got me out of the house and back into the real world. I was taking my time after six months of treatment for breast cancer – a lumpectomy, high dose chemotherapy with stem cell support and radiotherapy. My mind and my body needed time to recover. Life moved more slowly. Roy and I had built a new home, and we had a puppy.

That morning, things changed again. I had recently been to my specialist in Brisbane for another six-monthly check-up and everything was clear. Yet back in Canberra, a small node appeared in my neck. I had it tested. The earth shattered as my GP said, 'The cancer is back'. My body heaved with grief. I thought, this must be a nightmare. I could not believe what she was saying. I asked her to ring Roy for me and he was in her office, by my side, within minutes.

Back at work, the staff didn't know what I had been through.

'Has someone passed away?' Susie asked. It felt that way.

'The cancer that was in my body three years ago has come back.'

She couldn't believe it. 'You look so well,' she said. Words I had heard many times before.

Arriving home, our space of tranquility and peace, Max greeted us at the door; tail wagging as always.

Roy put his arms around me. We cried together. I held onto him; he was my strength, my hope, my inspiration, and my soulmate. We had another tough road ahead of us. My body shook with tears of sadness, tears of anger, tears of hopelessness.

This should not be happening. I married this man four years ago. There is no way I am letting go of him, and he will not let go of me either.

The bra!

The bra, or the brassiere; a woman's undergarment which supports the breasts (*The Pocket Macquarie Dictionary*). Also known as a boob tube, corset, over-the-shoulder-boulder-holder, it has been a part of a girl's life since her early teens.

I've always wanted to have pretty bra and undies sets. I can remember when my mother bought me my first bra; it was white cotton with broderie anglaise and had matching undies. How proud I was that day! A step towards womanhood.

I had always purchased matching sets. Having travelled overseas to France, Denmark, Switzerland and many other countries, brands such as Christian Dior and Yves St Laurent were part of my undergarment wardrobe. Back in Australia, Arianne, Elle Macpherson, Bendon and Bonds had also made their way into my drawer. Why was underwear so important to me? It made me feel feminine and sexy!

However, after a lumpectomy in February 2000, it was several months before I could wear my normal clothing or a bra again. By doing arm stretches daily, I slowly recovered normal movements in my arm and shoulder. My husband was so understanding and helpful.

After my second diagnosis and various treatments and medications, my weight went up and down, and my bra size changed with my body. Underwire bras were too uncomfortable. Instead I turned to sports bras and singlet tops with shelf bras. The sexiness had gone out of it.

I was telling my dearest friend, Amanda, how life had changed for me over the last three years. She suggested spending money on pretty corset-style tops without an underwire instead of on sports tops.

That day I emptied the top drawer of my dresser onto the bed. Out spilled all the bras I had not worn over the last few years. I shed a few tears for what I had lost.

But I am a woman and can still feel pretty and sexy! Thanks Amanda!

Afternoon tea

Dad had come to visit us on a hot Canberra day. It was December with not a breath of air.

I had breast cancer, Dad had prostate cancer. Both metastatic. It was as if we worked in tandem. I lay on the couch, trying to get comfortable, the pain gnawing away at me. Dad read the newspaper, also in pain. It was time for afternoon tea.

Two cups of Twinings Earl Grey, fine china and the pleasure that comes from a well-made cup of tea.

'Dad, would you like a cookie with your tea?' I asked.

He looked up with anticipation. 'Sure.'

I placed two cookies on a square china plate.

'Did you make them?'

I was always baking and usually had something in the freezer for unexpected guests, but I hadn't baked these ones. They were a gift from someone who cared.

Some time later, we sat there giggling like two school kids. The pain had drifted away, and even with the unbearable heat we felt some level of comfort and control. I had never before touched marijuana and here I was at thirty-six, with my sixty-six-year-old father, getting stoned!

My husband, downstairs in the garage working on his car, could hear us laughing and having the time of our lives. He knew neither of us drank much those days, so there was only one conclusion. Cookies! The story is often recounted at our dinner parties and barbeques.

Knowing that marijuana was decriminalised in the ACT in 1992 allowed me the freedom to 'have a go' without the fear of prosecution.

'The use of marijuana for medical or any other purpose is currently prohibited in Australia, although a process of law reform on this issue is current in New South Wales.' (*The Cancer Council NSW, May 2001*)

So, let's bake!

Trish Armstrong

All three hairs

In the shower
I noticed hair under my arms.
Uh oh. Will I look for
the shaver or the camera?
Will I document
this exciting event?
Or will I remove them,
the hairs,
all three of them?
I vaguely remember
the shaver was blue
with a wide sort of handle.

I have started a new
chemo this week.
My hair will fall out again,
all three hairs.

No hair for ten months.
Will I ever have hair again?
What do you do with hair?
Wash, dry, style, use product?
I don't even know anymore.

What lovely hair,
Everyone said.
What shiny hair.
'You won't lose your hair
will you?' they all asked.

What will I wear today?
A hat? There are
stand-by colours,
the navy or the cream.

A scarf? (choice of four).
They feel more comfortable
on my head
but slip around and off.

Or the *wig*.
I could wear the wig.
No. Admit that I have
no hair?
Admit to whom? Me.
Don't I know I have no hair?
But I have hair. Hairs.
Three of them.

Nemo

I spoke to a small boy yesterday at the post office
while I gazed at a cartoon picture of Nemo on the wall.
The boy told me he had the DVD at home
AND that he'd had it since before the film opened at the theatre
AND that he'd watched it lots and lots of times.
His mother took his hand and guided him towards the door
and left me looking at the cartoon with Nemo's picture on it.

And I remember. Snorkelling
in a world of magic
arms, legs moving, below the water
Fish quivering and gliding all around me.
Bubbles rising to the surface.

A drawer full of drugs

I sat in his office. The tests had been done. The biopsy results were in. No surprises. A mastectomy in two days. It was all right though. It was in the ducts and non-invasive, he said. He would do a reconstruction by muscle expander at the same time. He would cut off one and give me another! I chose to believe.

The operation was performed. The results were not as expected. The cancer had escaped the ducts and invaded a lymph gland. Don't panic. Have a course of chemotherapy and some hormone tablets. Have a mammogram once a year and physical checks several times a year.

Four years later, almost to the day, secondaries appeared. A pain in my back; a diagnosis of metastases in liver, lung and bones; a further diagnosis in my brain. I had not realised that any of this was even a possibility. I had been naive about breast cancer. I knew that I could get more lumps. I now know that I should have taken more responsibility. I must now be in control of my recovery.

This time I have taken it seriously. Secondaries. I have changed my oncologist. I am surprised at myself for having been so casual about the original breast cancer. Nobody volunteered information to me and I did not know what to ask. Other people were more frightened than me. They might have known where it could lead. They took the big 'C' seriously.

I am now on a strict diet, take many natural supplements, and attend doctors and healers who I feel help me. My chemo has stopped working and my oncologist has changed the combination of drugs. He says he has a drawer full of drugs to try yet! I am waiting for my next result, due in two weeks. I said I would not let waiting for appointments and results rule my life. But the relief when the results are good!

I wake up. I am so scared. I feel empty. I do not know where I am going. I want to be in control, but I am not.

The mouse

We are standing in the kitchen. My mother says, 'I have the weeding under control and I had a good game of tennis today.'

'My treatment is tomorrow,' I tell her. 'The drugs I'm on have stopped working. They're changing the combination.'

'I had another mouse in the house last night,' she says.

Hot

I sit in the sunshine
that bursts through
my windows
and I want
the heat
on me always.
I feel so cold this year.
I wear
layers and layers
of clothes.
I am thin.
I have lost weight.
How different
from last year,
before they played
with my hormonal
balance
and I was hot,
flushed
and damp.

Goodbye

The atmosphere in the room was hostile.
His family did not welcome me.
He lay in his hospital bed.
He was tired.
He did not have long.
I had come to say goodbye.
I leaned over the bed
and kissed him.
He had been good to me.

Judy Shepherdson

Daughter of mine

I tuck her into bed and she hugs me tight. I breathe in the innocence of my child, sweet like rose petals. Her little arms squeeze me as she burrows her head into my neck, her small body shuddering like a branch in a fierce wind. Our tears mingle and I stroke her long blond hair, waiting.

When her sobs subside, I hold her face in my hands and look into her almond-shaped eyes. Her arms are still wrapped around me. 'Mummy, don't go. I am so afraid you will go away and never come back.'

I take a deep breath and try to control myself. I shake. I feel like a bowl of jelly, bright crimson and all substance gone.

My daughter, the love of my life. What can I say? No words seem right. I climb into bed and hold her, never wanting to let her go.

We talk of beautiful flowers in a garden. I tell her that the people we love are like flowers – red roses, pink geraniums, yellow daffodils and purple irises – which bloom and then die. I tell her that some flowers bloom for a short time and others bloom longer.

I wrap her with my words in the colours of the rainbow, one soft shade at a time. And we lie together until her body relaxes, though her arm is still wrapped around my neck. Her breathing slows as she falls asleep.

I lie awake in the dark and curse this disease.

I watch and pray that I will see her achieve her dreams, grow, become a most beautiful woman, lover, mother, friend.

Hollow log

Wrapped in my doona I snuggle into a special place, my hollow log.

Six weeks I have been away from home. Six weeks of holding the pain deeply buried, having to pretend I was okay. Now, safe in my hollow log surrounded by my faithful four-legged friends, they comfort me; they ask no questions, I tell no lies.

I smell the earth brought in by a gentle breeze, hear the horses outside the window gnawing on grass. The heavy sound of their hooves as they wander. I bury my head. I feel like a dead log, dry and dusty, hollow and ready to splinter. I imagine I see the woodcutter, a vision from a childhood fairytale. With one swift hard blow I feel my head and body splinter; the tears are released. I let them come, tasting the saltiness. The screaming inside, buried, such sweet release to let go.

My breasts are gone. Breasts which nurtured and nourished four children. Breasts, which gave pleasure, made me feel sensual and alive. In their place scars, wounds, tapestry of the past ten years.

I mourn their loss.

The cancer has spread to my lung. I have travelled to a place I have no wish to be. The stakes have changed, the future more uncertain. Curtains are closed and I smell dust. Darkness. I don't want to come out of the hollow log.

Three days I hibernated in the log, nurturing and healing my soul. Not rising, not even showering, I remained in the moment, place of pain and grief.

Screams became sobs, tears began to dry.

My hollow log disintegrates and turns to mulch, thick, dark and moist. I wriggle along to find the light, allowing its brightness to enter my life. I breathe deeply and once again feel whole.

A duck for every treatment

*W*here are Daphne and Derek? I bask in the warm sun on my little verandah. There's a sound from around the corner of the neighbouring caravan. It's Daphne and Derek, the two black ducks who visit me daily.

This is a duck story.

I spied a tiny duck looking at me from a shelf – blue with purple-spotted wings. It was after my first radiotherapy treatment. I had stopped at an op shop and there he was, amid the wonderful clutter. I picked him up and closed my hand to keep him warm as he nestled in my palm. I decided that I needed a daily treatment duck to help me through this time.

My day did not start until I had found my 'duck of the day'. Treatment over, I went hunting and didn't go home until I had sourced a daily duck. Big ducks, little ducks, ducks of every colour and shape. In fact, some did not really resemble ducks at all. What a collection I amassed! All sorts of duck-like paraphernalia. Combing the eastern suburbs of Melbourne, some days I visited ten or more op shops before I found my 'duck of the day'. Ducks surrounded my life!

I was near the end of radiotherapy treatment. On a cold and wintry Friday evening my children and I sat together watching TV. The wind was howling but we heard a very faint tapping sound near the front door. My eldest son went outside to look, thinking perhaps one of his friends was playing a joke. He returned with his hands cupped together. 'Mum, look what I found.' It was a baby duck, soft, brown and frightened. A real duck had found me! I stroked his soft, downy feathers. What did this mean? We fed him bread and water. During the night I thought I could hear the mother duck's frantic calls, searching for her lost duckling. I did not sleep easy. The following morning the duck wandered around the house. We went to the children's basketball matches, leaving the duckling home safe and warm.

When we got back, I found my baby duck dead. I placed him in my hands, tried to will him back to life, to no avail. What does this mean? Am I going to die? I sat on the floor with the duck enclosed in my hands, crying. My children were hysterical. I must turn this around, I thought. I told them – 'Of all the houses to come to, this little duck found us. He came because he knew he would be safe and warm and chose to be here with us to die. We should feel privileged'. Together we buried the duck, then picked some red roses and white geraniums and placed them on his little plot of dug-up earth.

I continued to collect ducks until the end of my treatment. My large flock stayed with me for a year. After this time I put all of the ducks, apart from the first and the last ones, into boxes and returned them to our local op shop. They flew away for the new winter.

As I sit and write, I watch Daphne and Derek arrive. On the days I'm not outside, they sit on my front step and quack until I come out and feed them. They waddle along, gently quacking, their soft eyes and shiny silky feathers so close I can pat them. The ducks have found me again.

Hope and Crap

Once upon a time there was
a most beautiful teddy bear called Hope.
Gentle by nature, fluffy, cuddly, with wise brown eyes.
Hope was thoroughly spoilt and loved by all.
She travels to exotic places,
among celebrities and starlets
with outfits for every occasion.
Pink, everything is pink.
A dazzling pink ball dress, with glitter,
Hope shines like a star.
In her own photo album,
testimonial to worldly adventures,
she is Hope, for all who cross her path.

And there is a wicked sister, a twin.
She is pink, bright pink
with lime green hair standing on end.
Her bright green nose sticks out.
No, not a pretty sight.
Her name is Crap.
That's Crap!
She grins,
her mouth open and wide.
That's Crap.
But she has a heart for a tongue,
a heart for a tongue.

She must speak.
She must speak of love.
Hope?
Sometimes
there is just
Crap.
But she has a heart
for a tongue.

April Fool's Day

I lie on a cold bench, surrounded by machines and computers. Clicking, buzzing, lights shining in my eyes. Cocooned in a space capsule.

'Time for your tattoo,' he says. He looks at me with boredom and resignation. 'I want a rose, not a bright blue dot.'

Thus begins the story. I had reached five years post-diagnosis and my celebration would be a tattoo. April Fool's Day, anniversary of diagnosis and surgery.

Designing my tattoo. A yellow rose. Five petals and five leaves. A closed bud for what had passed and an opening bud for what will be. Placed on my remaining breast, my celebration. When I looked at my breast all I could see was my gorgeous yellow rose.

Nine years pass and my breast betrays me and needs to be removed. But what of my tattoo? I told the surgeon, 'I don't care about my breast, but I must have my tattoo. Please can it stay?' 'The scar on that side will be lower,' he said. 'I don't care.' And stay it did, my little tattoo. The bud is still open.

April Fool's Day ten years on. My plan is to have a tattoo for every five years of survival. An orchid this time, yellow and purple.

'Squirrel', the tattoo artist, etched the orchid on my left ankle. He wanted to know the story. 'Your next tattoo in five years' time – it and the champagne'll be on me. But only if you sing karaoke.' I promised Squirrel I'd be there and sing in five years' time. Especially if the champagne is on him!

Dutiful daughter

'Don't cry,' Mother said.
The dutiful daughter obeyed.
I wanted to say – 'Mother, cry with me.'
But we cry alone.
She came into my room one night,
And sat on the bed.
I wanted her arms around me.
'You don't know
what you have done to me,'
she said.
When she had gone,
I cried tears of anger.
I wanted to scream
'You don't know how it feels to be me.'

I am frightened of the dark
like a child, sleeping with the light on.
And Mummy can't make it go away.

She is afraid of losing me
I am afraid of dying.
The light burns brightly.
Light of life.
But who, I ask, who will comfort me?

Sorry

'I have written you a letter,' he said. 'But I am not ready to give it to you.'

'Did you write the letter for you or for me?'

'Both,' he replied.

I found the letter in my car.

Four pages and ten years of bottled feelings. I read the letter through my tears.

Only now that I'm gone can he say these things to me. It's too late. He loves me I know.

I needed him.

The hurt will not go. Too much has been done. Words said in anger.

The way it has been, I journeyed alone. He could not walk beside me.

Living together but so far apart.

No greater loneliness than this.

I acknowledge his pain.

You can never go back. Too late.

Why weren't you with me then?

Letter to the editor

I would like to comment on your recent editorial, and I wish to make the following points in regard to living with a diagnosis of cancer.

Firstly, being labelled as a 'victim' or 'sufferer' does very little towards fostering a 'positive attitude'.

Secondly, adopting a 'positive attitude' does not guarantee that you will 'beat' the disease.

Following diagnosis, we would all like to know that having a 'positive attitude' will enable us to 'beat the disease'. For some of us, despite the most positive attitude and best treatment available, the reality is that nothing will ensure that the disease will be 'beaten'. And the unfortunate, heartbreaking consequence for some is a sense of guilt and failure.

Attitudes implicit in your comments raise unhelpful questions: Have I contributed to the disease in my body? Am I responsible for the return of the disease? Have I done something wrong, eaten the wrong food, become too stressed? The implication is that despite all your best efforts, you have failed. These attitudes and the feelings that they generate are very destructive. Facing a life-threatening illness, who needs to feel the added burden of a lack of a 'positive attitude'?

Being positive is different for each of us. It may simply mean being able to rise up out of bed each morning – at one point in my life, that was all I could muster. Perhaps all you can do is spend time with your children, walk the dog, manage simple household chores or spend time in the garden.

For me, a diagnosis of cancer was not about developing a 'positive attitude', but about learning to accept and live with life's uncertainties. And it has taught me to appreciate each and every moment of every day, even the bad ones. To value family and friendships and take absolutely nothing for granted. To be continually amazed at the beauty of the sky: morning, noon and night. To be so thankful to see the sunset each evening.

The reality for me was not 'fighting the cancer' or 'beating' it, but accepting, acknowledging and moving along with my life. And cancer did return to my body, despite my best efforts, but I did what I had to do and moved on again.

If you feel tempted to tell someone recently diagnosed or facing a life challenge to 'be positive', you may have their best interests at heart. But consider that this simple advice does not allow for the expression of fears or 'negative' emotions, which is very important.

This highlights the importance of support groups. They can be a safe place to express fears and emotions which need acknowledgment, and to gain support from others experiencing the same journey.

Never be afraid to share a hug or lend an ear to someone in need. It works wonders, and is far more comforting than the phrase 'be positive'.

Maria Waters

Chocolate frogs

The challenge

The challenge is
to accept the diagnosis,
and play the mind games of the subconscious.

The challenge is
to stay positive,
as the cancer cuts another path into my liver.

The challenge is
to smile,
when my mouth is full of ulcers.

The challenge is
to gather strength,
as fatigue possesses my body.

The challenge is
to have faith,
when a friend loses her battle.

The challenge is
to fight back tears
at my uncertain future among loved ones.

Casting out

I sit on the old wood verandah of our holiday shack with the morning sun filtering through the majestic flame tree. Across the dew-covered lawn, the ocean gently creases the white shore. In the distance, my husband casts his rod from the jetty that stretches out to the horizon. The peaceful surroundings consume me.

Eleven years ago, my husband was there with me watching my oncologist read my file. As his kind face looked up, I felt my heart in my throat — more bad news. Calmly, the doctor explained that my situation was not good and we discussed the best treatment option. Walking back to the car with my husband, I was engulfed by anger. Anger at this disease and what it was doing to my body and my family.

Now, I will join my husband. Barefoot I jump onto the wooden steps. The ocean slaps gently against them. As I walk across the jetty, beneath me swims a large stingray, a local in this area affectionately known as Monty.

I sit with my legs hanging over the jetty, the warmth of the sun on my back. We bait our hooks, cast the lines into the vast ocean and wait for a bite.

Filtered sounds

I lie in the sterile hospital bed, the surgical gown,
unflattering, wrapped around me.
My body smells of antiseptic wash,
as I wait to be taken down to theatre.
Sounds from the busy corridor
filter in through the slightly open door.
Nurses' stocking-covered legs swish past,
dangling keys clinking together in step.
Morning tea trays slide and rattle
across the metal trolley.
These tiny sounds flit through my mind
until the huge thoughts
of the cancer advancing in my tiny body
shove them away.

Four miles away

The boat cuts a path through the water, leaving behind a white wash and sunrays dancing over the ripples. Salt water sprays into my face and the breeze is cool. Near the four-mile reef, Alan cuts the motor, we throw anchor and our small boat bobs up and down with the slight swell.

Not so long ago, I was too ill from chemotherapy. I would be left on the shore, watching Alan, James and David drive off, boat in tow, for a day of fishing.

Now I look back to shore, some four miles away, part of it all and enjoy the thought of catching the big one.

Not like any other day

*L*ike any other morning, the six o'clock alarm clicks on to the chatting breakfast show announcer. I lie in our warm bed, straining to hear the news that has unfolded during the August night. But my thoughts wander to what I face today.

Ah. The familiar clatter of a breakfast bowl placed on the kitchen bench, a teaspoon hitting the side of a coffee mug; my husband in the kitchen. It is time to drag my forty-two kilogram frame out of the warm bed.

I confront the bathroom mirror. I see a pale face strained with worry. A silk nightdress hangs loosely on my weak frame.

Today is not like any other day. I will go to hospital for a liver biopsy to confirm 'probable infiltration of the cancer into the liver'.

I feel physically ill. I am scared. Do I have the strength to face a negative outcome?

A moment of joy

Children run around the oval with balloons and streamers, young faces painted with their team colours, ribbons of green, gold, blue and yellow pinned to clothing flapping in the chilly September breeze. It is the annual primary school sports carnival.

Lining the oval, parents and grandparents unfold chairs and place checked rugs on the freshly mown lawn for younger children. Picnic baskets and eskies, all shapes and sizes, are scattered around.

I sit among friends, with yellow streamers in one hand and a cup of hot coffee in the other. I watch and cheer loudly as our two young sons, James and David, run in the day's events. The joy of seeing them cross the finishing line!

Their beaming faces approach me, their tiny hands clutching ribbons. My eyes fill with tears. I am simply happy to be alive.

With the diagnosis of advanced breast cancer, I cherish these moments and desperately want to share the future with my sons.

My mother

I lie on the striped lounge draped with a rug, cushions under my bald head. I watch the sun filter through the blinds of the games room and the rays pierce the crystal glasses on the bar.

Today I am depressed; the treatment is playing games with my mind. 'Life is not worth living.'

My mother, a small rounded woman, the foundation of our family, sits beside me.

'Snap out of it; you have come this far,' she says. 'I will not bury my daughter, you will bury me first.' Her voice is stern.

For a moment I am angry. How dare she put this on me.

Looking up, I see tears in her eyes. No more needs to be said.

We hug and cry together.

Toontown

Hawaii, Los Angeles, San Francisco. Our holiday destinations for three weeks.

The itinerary has been finalised, passports are in order and I have good news from my oncologist. Tumour markers are down and the CT scan shows no further growth. 'Condition stable; go on holidays. Don't forget to send me a postcard. See you when you get back.'

After being diagnosed with advanced breast cancer in '92 with a poor prognosis, I never expected to hear those words. We have only to pack our bags and board the plane.

One of my favourite places is Disneyland. As my family and I enter one of the make-believe worlds, we are greeted by a brass Mickey Mouse statue, standing tall on a three-tier water fountain. In the background is a colourful city. A mountain peers over the top, displaying the word Toontown. Walking the winding streets, we are lost in the crazy world of cartoons. Odd shaped buildings lean in all directions; some look ready to burst, while others have tilted chimneys on slate roofs. Windows, square, round and arched, sit crooked in the brightly coloured walls. Archways supported by leaning pillars invite you to enter the buildings.

Look! Pluto! We stand side by side. Alan takes a photo.

Walking deeper into the make-believe world, we come across an old oak tree covered in autumn leaves. A carved plaque nailed to the protruding roots displays the names 'Chip 'N' Dale', and acorns are scattered along the ground. Wooden steps lead to the open trunk and a light inside suggests the furry friends are home. Let us go and see!

Feeling the effects of my treatment, I need to rest. We sit at a small round table, shaded by a red, white and blue striped umbrella, sipping cold drinks. Like a young child, I scan the street looking for a resident. In the distance, the Mickey Mouse clock that sits upon the red gabled roof of Toontown's City Hall clangs, bangs and whistles the hour.

What else would you expect in Toontown!

Bronwyn Taylor

Chemo Carol

She glides in wearing leopard-skin stilettos, enormous gold dangly earrings and hot sienna lipstick, her mascara startling among the rest of us who have lost our eyelashes. She exudes health, the outside world and possibilities as she straps on her apron. No floral frills here. Her apron is a full frontal of Michelangelo's *David*.

'Morning everybody,' she cries. 'Cafe chemo is open for business!' We sit in furry beanies and lopsided wigs, trying not to look as Jean searches for a fat vein, our eyes closing as the Phenergen kicks in. Carol is everywhere at once.

'The scones look hard,' she advises, 'I'd try the lemon sponge if I was you.'

Fred shuffles in on his walking frame and makes it to the Jason Recliner. Carol floats over and tucks him in with a white cotton blanket. 'Your cheese and bickies as usual,' she beams, 'and two sugars in the tea?'

Each Tuesday the crowd becomes more familiar. Tiny Rose is determined to get to her fiftieth wedding anniversary. Her emerald eyes are beady and her grin conspiratorial. She pats my hand and wishes me well. 'Look how it's growing back so thick,' she says of my new henna-coloured hair. I know the mangy patch at the front really looks more like a paddock with a few old gum trees than a luxuriant forest!

Fred has brought in a quiz book. Rose's face lights up. 'Come on Fred,' she squeals. 'Give us a hard one.'

Fred frowns into his spectacles. 'Name eight parts of the body made up of a three-letter word,' he reads.

I kick off cleverly with 'hip' and Rose's face crinkles up. 'Bum,' she snorts. That's the signal to lose it completely. We chortle and chat. We joke and we jostle. We belong in this shared journey.

Rose's husband Tom is admiring Carol's new apron. She tells him tales of picking up her husband from the airport wearing nothing but a fur coat. Tom is turning fuchsia pink and frothing just a little at the side of his mouth.

Anywhere else, I would gaze upon Carol with her tight leather pants, flirtatious decibels and unending cheerfulness with a disapproving eye. But here in this room of travellers desperate for another month (dare we ask for another year?), she is brilliant. Carol knows exactly what we need.

It is life full on. We laugh together and admire the trees turning gold and magenta.

An inspired hospital designer gave the oncology wards floor-to-ceiling windows. We can look out and savour every change in the seasons. I've seen those liquid ambers lose their leaves seven times now. Something they do here must be right.

Carol rushes to put my feet up as I struggle with the chair handle. 'You enjoy that snooze,' she smiles and turns back to Fred and Rose.

Lemon butter

'Sleep,' my mother commands. 'It is the best healer!' I remain obediently under the frothy floral doona. My legs luxuriate against the soft cotton and my ears love rubbing on my favourite fat pillow, but my mind is bursting out.

I scrunch up my eyes to pretend that the sun isn't streaming in behind the velvet curtains. It is so exciting to be back in my own bed!

The novelty of hospital life was wearing thin after seven years of operations. The surgeon had tried, to be sure. I had the best room in the place. I was seven floors up and the agency nurses would gasp at the view stretching south to the bay and far over to Donna Buang. A couch for visitors and vases provided in a hurry. I'd seen enough to know that this was a Rolls Royce hospital room.

But why do they attach those impossible foil covers to every orange juice? And does every morning have to begin with the toothy nurse from Dunedin plunging a Heparin needle into your quivering tummy? And why, when you are compelled to sit in front of the television for three days, is there nothing on but a Peruvian frog special, *The Bachelor 3* or *Talking Footy?* And how is it that Great-aunt Maude, hippie Talitha and sour workmate Ian ALL turn up at precisely five minutes past four? I felt like a pyjamaed Parkinson, encouraging convivial chat meaningful and thrilling to all! Funnily enough, Aunt Maude was quite taken by the tahini bake recipe!

'Now you stay there,' murmurs Gordon. 'I'll take the kids to school.' He disappears and the door juts open. A school-uniform-clad body slithers in beside me. We touch heads and I turn to see my son beaming. The door opens again.

'How are you, Mummy?' I feel a long plait brush my cheek. I open one eye and see a bright smile.

'Those earrings are not for school wear young lady,' I smirk.

She grins. 'Do you want me to open the curtains?'

'Come on, it's time to go. Get in the car,' yells Gordon.

The curtains part and sunlight bursts in. The lemon tree outside the window is groaning with a bumper harvest. We watch as Matthew raises his half-eaten vegemite toast to his mouth and straddles his blue and silver bike all in one go. He grins and waves and is off in a flash.

Ben and Claire's voices trail out the door. I hear the car tyres crunch on the gravel drive and fade away. I snuggle down into the doona.

Cutlery noises mingle with the neighbour's washing trolley scraping along the path. A red wattlebird screeches from the verandah. I open my eyes a little wider and see that my plump daffodil bulb has burst open under the lemon tree.

Sleep in? I don't think so.

I think I'll have a giant bubble bath and then make three jars of lemon butter. It is so delicious to be home.

Pat Mathew

Lube Queen of Australia

_L_ast year my son had an interesting time coming through Customs on his way home from London. He had brought with him a one-year supply of the non-hormonal vaginal moisturiser, Replens, which is no longer available in Australia. Customs repeatedly questioned him about the product, what it was used for, and why a thirty-year-old male was carrying a large amount of it. In the end he lost his cool, thumped the desk and yelled 'It's for my mother. She's got breast cancer. And she's got a dry fanny. And she needs it!' He got through with no further problems.

Many women suffer from vaginal dryness and atrophy as a side effect of their breast cancer treatment. There are many who would prefer not to use the commonly prescribed oestrogen creams to deal with this problem, even though we are assured by most members of the medical profession that even for women with oestrogen positive cancers it is safe to do so. It is claimed that there is no, or minimal, absorption of the oestrogen in these creams. Perhaps this is so, though no one has been able to explain to my satisfaction how, if there is no absorption, these creams actually work. And even if it is true, it seems illogical to say the least, to be swallowing anti-oestrogen preparations on a daily basis, while applying oestrogen to the other end!

Replens is an effective alternative for me and for several others with whom I have discussed this issue, but it went off the market in Australia in late 2001. The company that imported it decided not to renew their distribution licence because they were not selling enough to make it a viable financial proposition.

They say they launched the product on the Australian market with a one million dollar advertising campaign, but who would take notice of such advertising until they had a problem?

It appears to have been mainly word of mouth among women that was responsible for the sales that did occur. Mention it to many health professionals, even gynaecologists, oncologists and oncology nursing staff, and they haven't heard of it, or they refer to it as a lubricant. In fact it is much more efficient than a lubricant. It contains ingredients which attract and retain moisture, and once the tissues are rehydrated, an application every third or fourth day is usually enough to maintain healthy vaginal tissue.

There appears to be a lot of confusion about the difference between a lubricant and a moisturiser. Imagine tissue in the atrophied vagina as resembling a prune. Slather that prune with lubricant and what you get is a slippery prune. But rehydrate that tissue and it can become a plump, juicy plum.

When I first began searching for alternative non-hormonal products, I received quite a few free samples. These arrived regularly for several weeks, usually in plain brown packaging. It wasn't long before the postman was giving me odd looks. Despite the exaggerated claims of many of these products, most of them were not much better than the standard lubricants available here.

Some of the advertising was entertaining, particularly for one based on the by-products of hemp used for paper and textile manufacture. Not only is there a plain gel, it also comes in a variety of exotic flavours. There's a low fat decaf cappuccino flavour – a great start to the day, while for late night decadence, blueberry or strawberry cheesecake would be just the thing. As my principal interest is comfort, this was interesting, but not quite my cup of tea!

When our son was coming home again this year he purchased enough product for a one-year supply for me and a friend. It was in the lead-up to the war in the Middle East, and remembering his hassles with Customs last time, he decided to send the essential supplies by mail. He divided it up into several parcels, and each one had emblazoned on the customs declaration sticker on the front *vaginal moisturiser for mother*. Once again the postman had cause for speculation.

One of my brothers is investigating the legalities of importing and distributing it. Given the number of women affected by breast cancer treatment, women with other cancers, and post-menopausal women in general, we reckon that once word gets around there is a potentially lucrative market waiting.

Given the sensitive nature of this subject, it is hard to gauge the potential market. I once tried to get a national survey off the ground, but because it is something that few people are comfortable talking about, and because oestrogen products offer an easy out, it was dismissed as *a Tasmanian problem*.

I reckon this issue is as big or maybe even bigger than lymphoedema. Once women started to speak out about their problems with lymphoedema, public awareness was raised. The medical profession was no longer able to shrug it off as an unfortunate but inevitable consequence of cancer treatment, or to brush it under the carpet or leave it in the too-hard basket.

At the very least, we should have a choice.

We have had several discussions about the best way to raise public awareness. Our daughter has reservations about methods suggested so far. She says given the likelihood of journalistic licence, sensationalism and the misconceptions about lubricants and moisturisers, the outcome could be very embarrassing.

She says if she ever opens a magazine or newspaper to see me proclaimed Lube Queen of Australia, I am immediately disowned!

Going to God

I got a letter recently from an acquaintance who wants me to go to Canada with her to meet God. It's a waste of time going to Lourdes, she said, because at the moment he's in Edmonton.

Not so long ago I answered the doorbell at half past ten in the morning to be confronted by another sad-looking acquaintance bearing flowers and fruit. She repeatedly expressed her astonishment that not only was I out of bed, dressed and walking around, but that I looked normal.

When Mum was diagnosed with ovarian cancer she decided to tell only her immediate family. She didn't want news to get around the neighbourhood as she felt that this would make her the object of curiosity, speculation and pity. Of course, despite her best efforts, word did get out and the rumour mill went into overdrive.

A few years after Mum died I was diagnosed with breast cancer. Based on Mum's experiences, we decided to be completely open about the diagnosis and treatment details. I reasoned that because Mum kept the information to herself, people made up stories, so surely being honest would short circuit this process.

It doesn't work that way of course, or at least not in small towns where you are well known. No matter how much information is available, the rumours continue, and some of them are real beauties. Miss any social event, and immediately you are written off as suddenly deteriorated, having only weeks to live, and probably confined to bed.

When a friend was diagnosed with uterine cancer ten years after her breast cancer, someone asked her husband how she'd known she had a problem. He replied that she'd been bleeding, and as he'd already said she had uterine cancer, he probably didn't think it necessary to specify where the bleeding was. Soon after this I was accosted in the street by a woman demanding to know whether my friend was as bad as she'd heard. I replied that that depended on what she'd heard, and was then told that my friend was supposed to have bleeding lesions all over her body.

Now and again some of the members of our local support group tell each other stories we've heard, and we are constantly amazed at the inventiveness of the storytellers.

There is also a large percentage of the population who seem to have an insatiable need for gory details.

'How are you?' they ask. Assured that you are fine, they will peer closely into your face and press the point. 'Yes, *but how are you really?*'

Depending on my mood that day, I either just repeat that I'm feeling well at the moment, or say something provocative along the lines of 'Well, I'm not dead yet.'

My husband Peter often deals with this situation by saying that apart from a bit of cancer, there's absolutely nothing wrong with me.

Don't you worry about that

*H*e swept into the ward, arms full of papers and long, lanky body festooned with mobile phones and pagers. A nurse scurried along behind him carrying yet more files.

When he told me that the lump he'd removed from my breast a few days previously was definitely malignant, I asked what sort of follow-up treatment was likely.

'Don't you worry about that,' he said. 'You concentrate on recovering from the surgery, and I'll decide about further treatment.'

'Yeah, well we'll see about that,' I thought. 'If you think I'll take that attitude lying down you can think again.'

He then patted me on the shoulder and patronisingly told me it was okay to go ahead and cry. 'If I could collect all the tears from my patients and use them to water my garden, I'd have the most beautiful garden in the district,' he said.

A couple of days later when I was preparing for discharge, another nurse came into my room and pulled a small piece of paper out of her pocket. She looked around then closed the door before handing it to me. There was a name and a phone number on the paper, which she said was the contact point for the Breast Cancer Support Service.

'But please don't tell him I gave it to you,' she said. 'He doesn't like his patients to talk to anyone else before he decides on their treatment.'

Of course one of the first things I did when I got home was to ring the number. By the time I went back to have the sutures removed I'd talked to several people, we'd read the literature provided by the Cancer Council, and compiled a long list of questions.

Peter put the clipboard on the desk, and we prepared to go into battle for information.

My first question, 'What sort of cancer was it?', seemed to surprise him.

'Breast cancer,' he said.

I felt like saying 'I know that you idiot. It's not part of my big toe that's missing,' but I quietly replied that there was more than one kind of breast cancer.

'Oh,' he said sarcastically. '*You've been reading books.*' 'Well,' he continued after a pause, 'I suppose you want a copy of the pathology report.' And he slapped a sheet of paper down on top of our list of questions.

He then handed me a referral to an oncologist and we left without asking any more questions.

'Ave a go…

I recently heard some men with prostate cancer asking for advice on ways to attract funding so that they could pay a professional to run their support group. They were astonished that we just did it, and wanted to know how we did it and why.

Many people, especially men, comment and complain about the publicity and the funding that breast cancer attracts. God helps those who help themselves, and women with breast cancer are living proof of this. But it's not simple.

We go all out to attract the publicity. We tell our stories in public, we speak to the media, we do all we can to raise awareness. We make our voices heard. There is strength in numbers, and it is very apparent how many of us are affected by this disease and how it impacts on the wider community.

We see a need, we have a go, we fine tune the process as we go along. We do it to help ourselves and to help other women.

Playboy centrefold

*I*f I'd ever secretly harboured the desire to be a *Playboy* centrefold, I've left my run too late.

When I had a lumpectomy in 1996, the surgeon removed about two-thirds of the top part of my left breast. When the wound was sutured together, this had the same effect as a facelift. My much smaller and neater breast was hitched up a good couple of inches, and now looks at the world with a jaunty air. The other one is showing signs of age, and has a definite fifties droop. When the surgeon made tentative enquiries about reconstruction, I told him that if I ever decided to have anything done, I'd rather have the other one pruned to match.

I have a crater where my armpit used to be (but on the up side it is now hairless), and a 'fat' left arm from lymphoedema.

The right side of my body is not unmarked either. I'm now onto my third infusaport. The first one was in too deep and was very hard to access, so I had it removed when I'd finished the first lot of chemo. The second port went wrong. It moved and pulled the catheter out of the vein, so it also had to go. Before the surgeon put the third one in, we discussed the previous problems. He decided that he'd do a little 'fat-ectomy' first, so this port is just under the skin. It sticks out like the proverbial knot on a log, and is surrounded by a tracery of scars. But it works like a dream.

Added to that lot is the tram track down the middle of my chest. In 2000 a second bout of endocarditis finished off my damaged mitral valve, so I had open heart surgery. The nice, expensive little valve ticking away in my chest sounds like the crystal clock which used to be on Grandma's dressing table.

In 2002, a series of very peculiar liver function test results led to many diagnostic procedures which finally revealed a tumour on the end of my common bile duct. Despite all odds, this tumour, although pre-cancerous, was not related to my breast cancer. However, the resulting surgery left a lovely scar right across the top of my abdomen.

Last year this monument to modern surgery was topped off

when I acquired Horner's syndrome. This means that I have a lopsided head, or to put it in polite medical jargon, an asymmetrical face. The droopy eyelid, contracted pupil, and out-of-alignment eyebrow are caused by nerve damage from the pressure of tumours in the lymph nodes of my neck.

Horner's is apparently more usually associated with metastatic lung cancer, but if you are looking for information on the Internet, it pays to be very specific in wording the query. As some breeds of dog have a genetic predisposition to nerve damage causing Horner's, there is a lot of interesting, but largely useless, veterinary information available.

The first time my hair fell out it grew back as thick as ever, and very curly. For a while it was like an afro, almost impossible to get a comb through. I had it cut several times before it eventually returned to manageable waves. The second time it grew back nicely wavy, but so far this time it has thinned dramatically and gone straight. The texture has changed though, and it is now a bit like straw. It would probably look good on a scarecrow.

When one of our granddaughters was visiting last week she was full of chatter about her friend Matilda. 'Me and 'Til are going to be a hairdresser,' she said. She climbed onto the couch and told me to sit forward so that she could stand behind me. Then she brushed and combed, primped and curled, and applied a vast quantity of imaginary mousse, gel, spray and colour before getting out the pretend make-up.

'Finished,' she said. 'Now I'll make you a 'pointment for next week. What day would you like?'

'Hang on. First I need a mirror to see if you did a good job. Do I look nice?'

'Nanny you look bootiful.'

I hugged her and thought that none of my battle scars are very important.

Lee-anne Hazeldene

The bald-headed beauty

A good friend of mine suggested I cut off my hair before it fell out.

It was long and dark and would grow back quickly, wouldn't it? It always did grow fast, and it was so thick. I sat on the chair as my hair was divided and then plaited. I wanted to save these braids for my two girls, and for me too.

'Are you ready?' Sue asked. My throat swelled.

'Yes,' I croaked. I felt comforting arms around my shoulders.

The snip was a chainsaw tearing off a limb. Then another snip and another. Then the clippers were switched on as tears slipped down my cheeks. I closed my eyes and tried to block out the sound. I felt like a sheep being shorn. When the noise ceased, I opened my eyes to reality. It was gone, my hair was all gone. Who was this person in the mirror?

Sue tried to comfort me. 'You have a lovely shaped head,' she said. Maybe this was true? Maybe now I'm a bald-headed beauty.

B1 and B2

*N*o, this is not a children's story. So what's with the name B1 and B2, you're thinking? Let the story begin…

As we entered the building, my stomach was churning and my nerves were on high alert. My girlfriend Anna gently held my hand. Our eyes met and no words were needed.

'Please take a seat and your name will be called shortly,' the receptionist said with a friendly smile.

I scanned the assortment of people. Some pale, sombre. An elderly couple sat frailly. Several others kept checking their watches, busy people in a hurry to be anywhere but here. I searched through the magazines sprawled across a highly polished table.

'I wonder how long this will take?' I whispered to Anna.

Eventually my name was called. I dropped the magazine, grabbed my bag. The nurse led me to a cubicle and asked me to sit there and wait to be called again. People went in and out of two doors opposite my cubicle. On one door was a sign, B1, and on the other, B2. Below that, in all their glory, were the Bananas in Pyjamas! At least someone here must have a sense of humour.

My heart beat rapidly as I followed the nurse into B1; radiology machine B1. The room was cold and smelled sterile. The radiologist asked me to lie on the bed and explained what would happen to me during each treatment.

'At this stage, you will be having seventeen treatments over the next four weeks. It will take about fifteen minutes to get you exactly lined up under the machine, then Michelle and I will go into that room behind you. We will be able to see and hear you the whole time we are in there, so if you want anything all you have to do is tell us. The actual radiation treatment only goes for about five minutes. Then we will come back in and you can go. Now, are you okay with all that?'

'I suppose so.' Just get this thing done and let me out of here.

I lay there with blue marks drawn on my head, taking deep breaths, trying to relax. I imagined that the rays were killing off any little cancer cells roaming around in my head. The machine buzzed loudly, then it would go quiet, then buzz again. Each time the buzzing went on for longer. My mind would wander, so I concentrated even harder. Those little suckers were being buzzed to death by B1, who was going to be my friend for the next four weeks.

How do you tell them?

I have always been honest with my children, but now I don't know what to do.

They were aged between two and nine when I was initially diagnosed. My eldest was worried that I would die, just like Granny, who had passed away two years earlier from leukaemia. I explained how my cancer was different and how Granny's was in her blood. 'They couldn't take out all of her blood and put in a new lot to get rid of the cancer,' I told them when Granny died.

It was not so hard to tell them about my tumours that could be removed. 'They will cut out the two lumps, then give me chemotherapy to kill off any little cells that were too small to find. Then I will be all better,' I told them when I was going into hospital to have surgery.

My youngest turned three when I had the lumps removed, and the next week it was Christmas. Fear of the unknown caused grief for all the people around me. For me though, the thought that I might die never really entered my head. I knew that I had to get better for my children. They were so young and innocent, still needing their mother's care.

The Christmas just after the mastectomy was special. Then I had chemotherapy for six months. I was lucky; I didn't have much nausea, just a feeling like morning sickness. But the tiredness! I could not believe someone could be so tired. Keeping up with three young children, a husband, a house and a business was a real challenge.

Over the next two-and-a-half years, my marriage broke down, I moved out of the family home and lost full-time custody of my children. It nearly broke me.

I began a new relationship with much trepidation. Then I was diagnosed with a tumour in my skull. I found out in the middle of my son's tenth birthday tea. So much for breaking it to them gently! Yet another bout of tears for us all.

This time I had twenty-five treatments of radiotherapy over a six-week period. I had to stay with friends in Melbourne during the week, but I would travel home each weekend to see my children.

I joined the nude-headed brigade after a few treatments. This was very painful to accept as I used to have long, beautiful hair. The tiredness was upon me again, but at least I didn't have the same hectic workload this time.

I struggled through the next two years. I had horrific bouts of depression, and once thought I should take my own life. I had a bitter ex-husband, a custody fight through the courts and a difficult teenage daughter. Things got rosier (ha! ha!) with the end of my eighteen month relationship. I did finally get to the end of my settlement though, so at least I had some money again.

I was at breaking point again, so I decided to do something drastic. Within three weeks, I had packed up my rented house and put everything into storage. My dog Ernie and I hopped in the car and travelled around Australia for three-and-a-half months. Then, in Mackay, three-quarters of the way around the continent, I was diagnosed with a tumour in my spinal column.

I flew home with Ernie so I could have immediate surgery in Melbourne.

I explained it all to the children, yet again, when they came to the hospital just before my operation. 'It's the same as before. They will cut the tumour out. They will give me radiotherapy to kill any little cells that might still be around. Then I'll be all better again.'

I didn't lose all my hair this time, but I think I lost a bit more hope. What if the cancer returned yet again? And I had that damn tiredness again.

Well, only one year on and bad news came again. Now the cancer has decided to take a different course and has leeched its way into my bones. Just saying it makes me feel the leeches covering my bones inside me.

I was angry, so very angry!

So what would I tell my children now?

Just a week ago, the doctors told me they had made a mistake. It wasn't in my bones at all. I could tell my children that.

My pack of cards

So who says life is fair? Sometimes life can be like a pack of cards. The ace might be dealt often, or you might be forever drawing twos. In life it often feels as though you are drifting somewhere in the middle, like a seven.

Six years ago I drew a two when I was diagnosed with breast cancer. I had a positive attitude and in no time I was back up there getting tens. Then I separated from my husband. I think I got a three that time. I started the climb back up to my tens, but the two popped up again when the cancer returned.

I was generally getting fives for the next two years, with some ups and some downs. Things can't get any worse I thought, but they did! That damn two turned up again; another tumour! Why me, why me? Just give me a break! Wasn't it my turn to draw an ace yet?

Oh no, a year on and I think I have the two of clubs; it's in my bones. This time it is different though. I've returned to my faith in God and the many prayers for me will be answered! There are no more twos left in the pack now anyway, so there's only one way to go and that's up!

I think, what I need now is an ace, but sometimes our expectations are too high.

The doctors have just told me that they made a mistake. It's not in my bones. A queen. What bliss!

The chocolate frogs

My oncologist had to pull a few strings. He was arranging my urgent surgery to remove a tumour that had been found in my spinal column. 'I owe you some chocolate frogs,' he said to the person on the other end of the line.

'Do you pay *all* your colleagues with choccy frogs?' I asked him. It made me laugh despite the turmoil of hearing that the cancer had returned.

I armed myself with chocolate frogs for my next appointment with my radiation oncologist. Sometimes you can feel intimidated by specialists, but not this time. She reassured me that even doctors are human as she laughed and laughed when I gave her the frogs. I had to see a neurology surgeon next. I discovered that he liked white chocolate frogs, definitely not brown ones.

My nerves were pulled taut as I was prepared for theatre. I cried and cried as I left my children and friends. As they wheeled me into the smell of the sterile theatre I asked, 'Is the surgeon inside yet?'

'Yes,' replied the nurse. I handed her two white chocolate frogs to give to him. A few moments later he appeared with a big grin on his face. We all laughed and laughed.

'Do a good job please!'

He placed his hand on mine. 'Yes, of course!' he said.

Lyn Clarke

BC Mets

'I have a really bad back,' I say, staring past the young lady doctor I have chosen because she has the same name as my best friend. I take a deep breath, because there is no point in coming here unless I screw up my courage to add '…and I have a lump in my breast.' The words catch as I squeeze them out. Has she heard? Yes.

On the examination table she kneads my underarm. 'Is there anything there?' I ask.

'I can't feel anything.' She starts kneading into my breast. 'Yes,' she whispers, eyes squinted in concentration, 'at least three.'

'And the breast?' I manage, 'You think it's cancer?'

'Oh yes,' she says. 'No doubt in my mind.'

I breathe in and gather my courage, but I never get the question out. No matter; she sees and understands.

'Two years,' she says, 'But some do better. What are you doing for the pain?'

I mumble about codeine and Nurofen and she nods and believes me. I wish she could read my face again and help me without my having to ask.

'You'll need to see a surgeon very quickly,' she says.

I start to cry. 'Isn't it too late?' Tears plop down my face and I look around the room and realise there are no tissues. My nose starts to run and I purse my mouth shut. Great! She leaves.

She comes back with tissues but I have already used my sleeve.

'The surgeon is just your first stop. She'll advise you on what will happen,' she says looking across the table at me with newly sad eyes. 'You'll need a doctor. I'd like to be your doctor.'

I knew once I came here and told I would be on a rollercoaster.

'I'll be there for you if you choose me. At any time during this journey, if you need me.'

Journey. It's the first time I have heard the word, except about trains and planes and buses.

She hands me books and brochures and sticky notes with

phone numbers on them. I clasp it all to me and stand up without shaking. I leave the room and the building and strap myself into the second last car of the biggest roller-coaster I've ever seen.

I'd like to call the roller-coaster something that is exciting and a bit out there. How about 'BC Mets'?

Talking on Tuesdays

*I*t's Tuesday, so I do what I always do on a Tuesday. I get up and take my morphine and, to ward off the dreaded constipation, its 'sad little mate', coloxyl and senna. I shower and rub on the cream that has almost vanished the horrific burn I copped from the radiotherapy. I dress and make sure I don't forget to pop in my tit. Too often at work I have looked down and – whoops! Fly back to the car and the house for the prosthesis. I do the face and eye creams and the make-up. I give the wig a spray of water and a few shakes before I put it on. Then I am at last ready for the world.

At work it's business as usual. I don't lift anymore, but that is my only concession, and the only one made to me by my workmates. But this is Tuesday.

On Tuesdays I turn my phone to divert for an hour and talk with twenty other women who have also taken the morph, donned the wig, crisped up with the radiotherapy and dreaded the chemo. I can speak with others who know it's there in the bone or the lung or the liver or the brain or any combination of the above. Women who understand that they will probably not get well from this scourge. Friends who have cancerous bones steadied with steel and tumorous kidneys bypassed with surgery. People for whom an ache in the foot means 'Oh shit, I need some radiotherapy', and after a bone scan result dig out the sick bowl and the bandanas. Sounds hopeless and helpless. It's not.

In those first dreadful months, I realised in my rare lucid moments that I craved contact with women who were also dying from the same bitch that had somehow snuck up on me. Instead, I found myself surrounded by women who were living with it. Their routines were interrupted by treatments, medical appointments and setbacks, but their lives went on and were rich and wonderful. I had never imagined that.

So on Tuesdays we talk about medication and husbands and government policies. We read with envy postcards from those of us who are in France or Turkey. We chat about the mundane and mention the unmentionable. Most of all, we acknowledge and celebrate the fact that there is life after a diagnosis of metastatic breast cancer.

To this group I bring all the questions and sadness that my dear loving family could never come close to understanding. From this group I gain answers and ears and tips, but most of all, the knowledge that I can live on and contribute to this wonderful world of which I am a very special part.

The hour goes so fast and the business calls start again, but Tuesday is the one day when I know my heart will be enriched and my spirits lifted, thanks to our group.

Girlfriends

*S*tand back Thelma and Louise. Let's hear it for Doris and Beryl, the forty-somethingish pair who have known each other since kindy and holiday together every few years despite the half-a-world that separates them.

We worked in a plug factory at seventeen to pay for our dream escape. Production line boredom was worth it as we jetted off to boys and Benidorm, Spain and sunshine. Remember the beery louts we fought off with their sure fire chat-up lines? Remember those we didn't fight off as the dry dusty sunshine crept through the tall windows and onto the terrazzo floors?

I laughed at your terrified expression when we chose a deserted Queensland beach hut with possums curling in the rafters and spiders you could hear scuttling in the toilet.

And Prague. Oh, how I longed to polish every copper-topped building, and you wanted to take home every thin, grubby, gypsy baby.

In 2002 it was Tasmania. Meeting in Sydney, we glanced at ourselves in shop windows. We could not see the penniless students or the naive young women we had been. We ate upmarket and chose hotel suites for the view and the spa and set off for Hobart with more clothes than we had packed.

Gradually, we ticked off our list of 'must-do's'. We bushwalked for days, turning dusty well-trodden corners to be confronted by the crashing cliff-faced coastline.

We surrounded ourselves with purple and lavished ourselves in lavender. We trekked miles to sit beside a giant waterfall. Years before, we both lived beside highways. We used to drift to sleep imagining the traffic noise was a waterfall crashing down. We closed our eyes and drifted back.

Then, with the holiday over, I came home. I showered, put my arm up to apply deodorant and there it was. A strange dimple, but no lump. My hand flashed to my breast. There was a lump, but so small it was nothing. The heady smell of lavender was overpowered by my confrontation in the bathroom mirror. Our holiday became a time frame and my life became a roller-coaster.

More power to Doris and Beryl.

Let's salsa in Peru and scuba in the Caribbean.

Let's go to our high school reunion in platform shoes and false eyelashes and pity all those who lost their best friends along the way. Because we didn't.

My sister

*M*y sister is the cleverest, funniest person I know.

She was born when I was a spoiled two-year-old. They have told me the story so often I think I remember pushing the chair to the front window and climbing up. I shouted out to every passer-by, 'I've got a baby sister and she's got black hair just like my dad and I'm going to call her Jolly.'

She was born at home. She was born in my single bed with the mauve wrought iron. They took me in to see her. There was Mum holding the bundle with the black hair spiking out at the top. Closer. She was tiny and her eyes were slanted and her lashes were thick and dark.

I loved her from that moment. They called her Jolie. We grew and became people. Me, the shouty attention grabber. She, the quieter, more sombre plodder.

When I was thirteen our father died. I screamed and became hysterical. My grandparents reached for me and wept as they squeezed my arms. I threw myself on the floor and aunts scooped me up and held me crushingly close while uncles pressed glasses of whiskey to my lips.

She sat quietly to one side as tears welled through those thick black lashes. She was eleven.

My sister is the cleverest, funniest, meekest person I know.

By sixteen I was wild and dangerous. Mum waited up all night for me to come home. I bothered if it suited me. The family sat me down and chatted. I nodded and smiled and planned my next big night out.

She just went to school. She slipped in and out of the house at reasonable hours and scuttled for cover each time she heard yelling in the kitchen. She was fourteen.

My sister is the cleverest, funniest, meekest, truest person I know.

Then I got pregnant and came to Australia. She became the only child. She was sixteen.

My sister is the cleverest, funniest, meekest, truest, craziest person I know.

She dressed in gorilla suits and dashed through maternity wards yelling 'I've got to push.' She became a stripagram and a nurse and a midwife. Suddenly she was a mother and a wife and a homemaker.

I had captured the family's attention with my escapades. She earned it with her wit and tenacity.

Then at forty-five I got breast cancer.

She came and wheeled me down for radiotherapy on the tumour on my spine. She shaved my legs and painted my toenails and plucked the hairs around my nipples. She looked at me with so much love through those lush dark eyelashes. She was forty-three.

My sister is the cleverest, funniest, meekest, truest, craziest, and most wonderful person I know.

Bosom blues

I despised my breasts when they arrived, so big and bouncy on my small frame. I was so jealous when each bloke I'd fancy would rather talk to them than me. I hated them for each dress I couldn't carry and for each miracle of engineering that I called a bra which cut into my flesh and gave me blisters. I planned vengeance when the heat rash under them was red and bleeding and my back ached. I cursed them for every bikini I couldn't wear and every sport I looked silly playing. I forgave them.

I forgave them when plump little bodies suckled there, falling off, full as a goog, little rosebud mouths all milky and open. Little bodies, growing so quickly, nourished only by my breasts. Little fat bodies learning to be careful and not bite. Getting their little mouths ready to make names for the special stuff in my shirt. 'Nuck Wom' and 'Bo Bo' – my gift to my children that my wonderful breasts allowed me to give.

The children are all fine and grown now. Nuck Wom and Bo Bo went from some surgeon's bucket to the incinerator.

It's twelve months after my diagnosis with metastatic breast cancer. To my breasts, wherever you are, I did forgive you for being what you were all those years ago. I learned to love you for what you gave.

It's just that – fuck me – then you gave me this.

Promises

I once was the most educated person about breast cancer you could ever meet.

Ten years ago I saw my beloved mother-in-law touched then felled by this sneaky silent stalker.

I had promised her in tearful conversations in her dark dingy bedroom that I would check my breasts each month a week after my period. I would be alert to any change, any bleeding from the nipple, any lump or thickening.

I helped and tended her through the ice-cream-bucket-in-the-back-of-the-car days. I washed her when the lumps stopped the soap as I gently tried to guide it across her poor crippled back. I trudged the paths of the palliative care facilities with her, one every two days, because she knew she didn't have enough strength to do it all at once. She said that *he* would not be able to take care of her. She had promised *him* that in the end she would take care of herself because she knew *he* didn't have the bottle to do it.

In the end she was in the hospital.

In the end she was pleading for them not to take her to a place where you die.

In the end he took all of her day clothes home and put them in the bin. She cried and said that she had no strength to fight it anymore.

He spoke to his girlfriend on the phone, promising that it would not be long until they could be together, while Hazel lay hearing and hurting.

In the end all the promises were for naught.

My darling Hazel died in the hospital.

He turfed his lush of a girlfriend.

And I have breast cancer.

So much for promises.

I looked at my husband

I looked at my husband tonight,
jumping forward in his armchair, his face
illuminating, as his favourite footy team
flashed their blue and gold across the TV.
Beer at his side, fag ever in hand,
turning his urgent eyes to me
in the hope that I will
share that utter bliss.
Twenty-six years of togetherness
and we've shared almost all of it,
but not this.
Never the beery, blokey, footy-type passion.

Thank you my darling for sharing
all the wonderful riches.
The children, all six of them
out there making choices.
The business born of your dreams
but precious in my waking time.
Best marks though, for sharing
my recent nasties so well.

You move to the edge of your seat,
with the best yet to come,
and I can't wait.

Mary Dewhurst

The beautiful jumper

Leaving the chilly winter evening with its biting winds outside, I walked back into the casualty room at Armidale Hospital. It was six o'clock, Monday 29 April 2002.

The look on the young doctor's face told me that something was terribly wrong. My gut feeling all along had been that the breast cancer had travelled to the liver. Yes. He confirmed my suspicions. The room was surreal with a distant cacophony of sounds. Trolleys clanking, children crying, a woman in the next booth vomiting her heart out, pagers bleeping. People moved around me in a blur, with no shape or form. I held tightly to my young grandson's hand, my patient little man, who had been with me the whole day as I was propelled from one test to another. We held it together until our taxi pulled up at his home and my daughter ran towards us. All three of us huddled in the dark on the front lawn and cried and cried. Thus began my second journey with breast cancer. After treatment – hormones then chemotherapy.

Cancers, in the bones and in the liver, have now stabilised and I feel well.

Looking back, I remember feeling so out of control. The cancer was dictating and running my life, throbbing away in my liver and gobbling at my bones.

I had my hair shaved in the third week of chemo. This was my first act of taking control. Up until then, my hair had been falling out in chunks in the shower and going up my nostrils as I turned over on the pillow. I took a big breath, and said 'ready' to my hairdresser Pauline. After the deed, there were plenty of comments from the peanut gallery: 'You look good, Mary!', and, 'You'd do really well in saffron robes with a begging bowl on the corner of King and George Streets!' It lightened the atmosphere.

I remember other things. My whole body flushing, which happens when I am distressed. People discussing investment and retirement, and thinking, does that include me? Do I dare dream that I will go beyond stats?

My new Rubenesque figure was billowing, courtesy of the steroids I was taking as part of chemo. Would it be extravagant to go ahead and buy that soft, dreamy, beautiful jumper I saw yesterday? What if I buy the jumper and don't get good use out of it? Not enough time? My cancer friends and I always have a good chuckle when we have discussions like this. Peering over our cups of skinny chino and soy decaf latte, our eyes squinting, mirthful and knowing.

And now? I think I have grown; I am not the same person – my body, my perspectives and my priorities have changed. I have moments of darkness, but moments of bliss, joy and laughter too. Most importantly, I have kept doing the things on my Must Do List, which I keep adding to and enjoying.

My conversation with God

I sat in my fluffy lined cane chair being amused by the cheeky bower birds tossing pegs from the basket. The lilting sounds of Enya wafted through the doorway. The sweet scent of jasmine and freesias blended with the warm breeze. It was a delicious spring afternoon and I was at one with the world. But I needed some answers from God. I said: 'God, I need to talk with you right now.'

'Go right ahead,' God answered. 'I'm here all the time.'

I said: 'God, I should be damned angry. The house is paid off after years of blood, sweat and hysterics. Howard and I are not as money-challenged. There's my daughter Mel. My grandchildren, three precious little souls that I want to feed green lollies and red cordial – only joking God. Why do I have cancer? And twice at that?'

'Some people need a wake-up call,' said God. 'And twice at that! Aren't you taking time to enjoy the fruits of your labour these days? Isn't time with your family more special? By the way, how was your foodie weekend in Melbourne?'

'Good, God! Yes of course. But I want more time, a lifetime. I want to see Zakk, Dakota and Jacinta as teenagers giving their mother hell like she did to me – oops, sorry God. Being flippant again! I would like to see them as young independent adults. And there's Howard and me. Wouldn't it be nice if we could sit across the dinner table together in our twilight years and gum our food to death? And there's my little three-legged mate Zeus, who badly needs to see a doggy orthodontist. Who's going to love him more than me? What do you have to say about that?'

God answered: 'Mary, you may or may not do all that. How long do you want? What is a lifetime, anyway? Is it measured in years or quality? Some people are dead before they die. Mary, when your time comes, all will be well.'

'Mmmm, I'll think about that,' I said. 'Thanks God.' The warmth of the sun had enveloped my body. A bird whisked past my ear and I turned to see it fly the whole length of the verandah.

This is what I want to tell him

Let's forget about Jane's swanky afternoon tea. I don't want to suffer hours of verbal masturbation with her upwardly mobile friends.

We'll get rugged up in our winter woollies. Pack a thermos of hot, strong coffee. Take a few slabs of pastrami sandwiched between thick slices of rye with dill pickles. And then we'll head for our favourite spot at McCrossin's Mill beside the old wooden bridge. Let's see if Mildred and George have had signets yet. Heathcliffe will surely be glad to see us and greet us with a quack.

Techno symphony

The trolley with Caroline attached was hurtling towards me. I adjusted my back and bottom well into the Jason Recliner. 'Here we go again,' I thought.

My eyes had become heavy from the pre-med, but I was now on full alert, watching Caroline deftly preparing the gauze, tape and line. A second nurse appeared to do a double check and asked me, 'Your name is…?' I told her. But I have been coming here for a year; you'd think they'd know me by now!

There was much pumping, slapping and prodding of the back of my hand. My poor tortured veins were trying to hide from this cruel creature. Caroline called out, 'Sharp prick!' I looked to see if she was addressing Richard. When I turned back, she had the line secured and attached to the monitor before my body had the pleasure of tensing.

By the time I adjusted my pillow and blanket and made myself nice, the trolley had already led Caroline back to the prep room.

Nothing to do but to close my eyes and drift into noddy land.

Later, monitors called for attention, waking me as they built into a techno symphony, bleeping in unison. Occasionally one would break in and perform a solo. Then one by one, as if directed by a conductor, they made their exit. Until the last performer…then none.

Rejoicing

*W*aves darted in to tickle my feet as I strolled along the beach of the island. The warm breeze gently brushed at my sarong, caressing my freshly showered body. It was a new day and there was not another soul in sight. I danced and danced, pirouetting and leaping at the edge of the waves, rejoicing in my youth, good health and life itself.

I could smell food and hear sounds of the island and its inhabitants awaking; exotic aromas of nasi goreng wafting from the resort's kitchens, distant tinkling of glasses, someone coughing.

I allowed the fine white sand to run through my fingers once more before I sauntered up the narrow pathway to my bungalow, barely visible, secluded among the palms and frangipani trees.

The essence of Mary

tepping out of the bath, I caught a glimpse of myself in the mirror. I flipped Zeus off the edge of the towel and wrapped it around my body to hide it, thinking, 'Mary, that doesn't look like you.'

I stared defiantly into the mirror again. The hair is still growing, very short, very butch. Maybe I should go and buy a pair of Doc Martens to complete the look. My body, well, it's got more rolls than I care to have. And then there's the face. So fat and rotund that I could compete with Bert Newton for the title of Moon Face.

I don't recognise the new me at times, but I need to be kinder to myself and realise that the essence is still the same.

Jenny Morrison

In the bones

*H*ow could I not know that breast cancer could travel into my bones?

I am shocked that I, an educated woman who wanted to be so well informed about my condition, could not recall being told this by doctors. If I was told, I would most likely have recorded it in the little notebook I have taken with me to consultations with doctors over the last six-and-a-half years.

I reflected on my consultations with the surgeon I saw regularly after my lumpectomy. Our conversations were brief, efficient, elegant; I do not recall the detail. I do recall however the non-verbal, the physical, communications in the examination room – undo the buttons of my blouse and off with it, both breasts examined, arms extended in particular ways, glands checked. 'Thank you, that's fine, Ms Morrison.' Nothing non-verbal to hint at future changes in my skeletal system. I trusted this man, and still do. His non-verbal communication spoke of breasts only, breasts only. Maybe some soft tissue.

I was bewildered with my own lack of knowledge. I became a woman with a mission, a super sleuth!

Two things intrigued me:

Did other women know it could progress to their bones?

How did they learn this?

Wherever I went I asked these questions: at conferences, while camping beside the Pacific Ocean at 1770, on the Gold Coast, in Brisbane, Sydney, and Melbourne, on Lady Elliott Island while snorkelling, in Central Australia, at Hamilton Youth Camp and in the Yarra Valley. I found a cross-section of women living full and productive lives.

We would describe our common and not so common medical histories, and laugh and cry at our shared experiences. Then I went into sleuth mode: 'Do you have any recollection of your doctors telling you in advance that breast cancer can spread to the bones in the future?' or, 'How did you learn it had spread?'

Not one woman I have spoken to on the eastern seaboard of

Australia recalls being told of it as a possibility. Most (but not all) learned of it when they had hip and/or back pain.

Of course, I asked my doctor. 'How come I don't recall being told that breast cancer can travel to the bones?' That was met with thoughtful silence. Then, 'I expect I did tell you Jenny. It's so common.'

The next step was to talk to doctor friends and acquaintances. A more open question, over coffee or drinks. Almost universally, they would exclaim, 'But Jenny, you would have been told. It's just so common!'

My findings to date? Not one woman can recall being told that breast cancer can progress to the bones. I must add however that there is no method to my enquiries. I have just asked whenever the opportunity arose. Not a particularly valid research method it's true, but satisfying and enthralling!

And my conclusion? This does not mean we were not told. It could mean that information was provided by the doctors but NOT received or understood by me, or by other women. (Note my cautious approach!)

There is an easy remedy for this. We must ensure that doctors inform us in advance, at some early stage, of the potential progress of our disease. Tell us that the cancer could go into the bones, as well as to other regions. We need this information. Of course, timing is a critical factor, requiring careful judgment on the part of the doctor.

Also, progress to the bones, as a symptom of advancing disease, should always be mentioned in pamphlets, newsletters and other material available for women with breast cancer.

As for you, dear reader, please assist me in this campaign and the process of educating doctors and health professionals. Suggest to them that women should be informed that breast cancer can progress to the bones as well as to the breasts and other soft tissue!

Feel it

It was Ben who got me into all this. I loved Ben. Half my age, king of the pool. Coach of the university squad before work. Three lanes of ageing swimmers. Each of us felt Ben was our own individual discovery, a treat, like licking an ice-cream before work.

Ben was always on time. Six in the morning. Ready and waiting. We all loved Ben and we'd follow his program. We'd do anything he asked. Three groups – fast, medium and slow. And yes, I was the slowest in the slow lane. But did I learn to swim! I learned to train in the methodical way of elite athletes.

I finally asked him, 'Ben, what's the key to all this?'

'Just feel the water, Jenny. Just feel it in your hands and pull, slowly. That's what it's all about.'

And so I felt the water cross my body and held it in my hands for nine years. I loved the sense of control and power my body had. It could do anything as I swam lap after lap, year after year, pulling with my arms, driving with my legs. Then I was diagnosed with secondary breast cancer and it all changed. So now I will water walk. At least, that is my plan.

Water walking

I wander into the university pool. Hot, hot day with strong north-westerlies blowing the leaves and dust. Just here to look. Not swimming this time. Dressed in slacks and T-shirt, joggers on my feet. No togs and towel. Not confident any longer. My breathing feels shot to pieces, I have oedema in the base of my lungs. Consequently, my ribs and diaphragm are strained after the short walk from the car. My arms have that flabby old woman look which fascinated me when I was a child.

I sit down. Eight lanes – about thirty swimmers in all. Gum trees bloom along the fence line. Lean bodies lie absorbing the sun. Books. Papers. Some pretence of study. I look at the lane I used to swim in. Lane two. Not lane three or seven, which I used when I was a *real* swimmer. I made choices when I was well and swam two kilometres a day.

Lane two came after the diagnosis of advanced breast cancer, after chemo, after radiation; it came when my body was no longer my own. Lane two is the rehabilitation lane, divided in half to create two lanes of twenty-five metres. The effort is not the same as fifty metres, and the staff can see those of us with injuries and health problems from their office. No one in lane two yet. The sun is still low over the hills on the other side of the river. The water is smooth, the sun slicing through as it continues its slow ascent. The bottom is clean as always, despite the wind.

I'm heavier now – thick waist, not much strength. Will my togs fit? Will someone keep an eye on me? Five minutes of slow water walking is all I want, just to be in the water and look around, just to be in charge of my body again. I wonder if I can do it. Water walking is great. You select a belt made of dense polystyrene to keep you vertical in the water. Compressed around the ribs and the back, you adjust it to your waist, wander to the ladder and climb down.

I feel the cold so much now. Or is that my imagination? Stop procrastinating. Just do it. Come back soon. Five minutes will be enough, then build from there.

Fun? Fun!

Enough of this nonsense. I drive the short distance to the university pool. Summer's here. A hazy blue sky, no clouds, some light dust on my teeth. No more excuses. I pull into the disabled park beside the pool. I can walk. I just can't carry things for any distance.

I get my carefully packed rucksack out of the boot. Towel, sun factor thirty, sorbolene cream. I no longer need the hair brush. I put on my hat, bought on a hot day in the Sydney Botanical Gardens – cream on top, green underneath. It's like an old habit. I only wear it water walking.

I walk in, purposefully this time. I wonder who is on the gate? Great staff here, welcoming of all ages and stages. It's Jenny, a tall former Olympic swimmer with long blond hair. She is in charge of the Learn to Swim classes.

'Jenny, you're back.' She smiles.

'Yes,' I say, 'Big year.'

'So I heard.' She continues to smile.

There are kids everywhere, particularly in lanes one and two. Must be school holidays. I feel sick in the stomach.

'School holidays Jenny. You'd better have lane three. No jumpers,' she says. 'You'll be right. We'll keep an eye on you.'

I plonk my stuff down on a seat among the round tables. I have a plan, a no-nonsense plan. I've put my togs on at home. They still fit me. I've covered my face with sun factor thirty. Take off the T-shirt, take off the shorts. Joggers and socks. Collect a water-walking vest. Go to the ladder and get in. That's the plan.

I don my hat and sunglasses. Go to the ladder. Kids everywhere. Jump, splash, yell. 'Come away boys,' their mother calls, 'Give her some space.'

First foot down, followed by the second. Water at my knees. Coldish. Another foot down. Water at my thighs. The boys look at me curiously. I look at my knees. I freeze. 'You okay, love?' asks their mother. I nod. Big breath. Down another step. Let's get this over.

I kick away and head across to the third lane, pulling myself over the lane dividers.

Now it's on. No more nonsense.

Left arm out, right leg. Pull gently. What a relief. Right arm out, left leg stretched. Pull gently. Feel the water. Adjust my silly hat, sunglasses and the water-walking vest. I note the time. Ten thirty-five. I head for the shallow end. Slowly, slowly, stretch out my hands. Stretch out my legs, right out behind me. I feel the water lap across my breasts. Coldish. Just a little more effort will help. I pull with greater strength. Stretch out more. Again and again. Knees up and down but with a long gentle kick out the back. This is so great! Feel the water. I can feel the water after all.

Now I can look around. Blue sky, no clouds, clusters of white fluffy balls on the gum trees – just as it was last year, and the year before, and the year before that.

I'm nearly at the shallow end. A young woman is resting her face on her arms across the concrete wall. She turns, looks at me and laughs. 'That looks like fun. Is it?'

Is it fun? I think a minute. 'It's just great – feeling the water. It's so much fun!'

Ace

I stand, tennis racquet in hand, foot parallel to the baseline. Queensland sweat pours down my arms, across my lips. I lick them. Salty. I bounce the ball twice – slowly. Eyeing off the opposition. Solid man, strong forearms. Rod Laver type with ginger hair.

I hold the ball to the racquet, line up the spot, bounce it again. The thrill of it.

Here comes the toss. Up it goes. White ball, up, up, ever so slowly, completely controlled. My racquet is behind it. My feet come off the ground. The ball drops slightly. Then, thump – solid, firm and centred. What a sense of power. How I love that feeling!

I hit it. Fast. Right on the centre line. Untouchable. An ace.

That's how it used to be.

Nothing like it

I have been growing bush orchids for three years, since I learned that my cancer has spread. I want to do things. Sometimes even reading is difficult. It requires concentration.

So, I look after my bush orchids. I separated them from a large plant at my mother's place, gently planted them in orchid chips, and willed them to live. 'Live, grow and flower,' I would say to them as I tended them through the first year, then through the second and now through the third.

Today I went out and looked at them on the patio. Many plants in three plastic containers. They tell me that the flowers grow from stalks. I have nine stalks that reach boldly out to the sunlight, tall and elegant. They just keep reaching, gently stretching and erect. They are almost as tall as me. In one container though, the stalks are only waist high. Maybe I should have staked them as my friend Kris suggested. I am not a gardener. Where would I get stakes?

How does one stake plants? What do I do about these curves and bends? Where will the flowers come from? What are these thickenings? I inspect them daily. Grow, please grow.

I struggle to make use of time in a different way. I'm not the task-oriented person that I once was. I wait for the flowers.

'They will flower within the week, Jenny,' says my friend Kris. She knows about these things.

A flowering. My accomplishment of the last three years! I look again for the swelling as the buds enlarge, hoping they will flower before I go to Yamba. I am going boating and fishing for a month and I couldn't bear it if they flowered in my absence.

Plans must be made. One plant can come in my friend Pam's tiny car. Kris will come the second week and she can bring one too. My mother can have the third plant to enjoy. I particularly want to give her this as her health has prevented her tending her own plants. They look as though they may well die.

And so I continue to wait for the blooming. I have waited year after year, week after week, day after day. Perhaps at Yamba.

Gayle Creed

Walks with Seiko 115

Chocolate frogs

Walks with Seiko

I love her and she loves me. For the past twelve years Seiko and I have been constant companions. The bond between us is powerful and not fully understood.

Her cataract-clouded eyes shine green in the light these days, but she can still sense when I am in need of her. The love simply radiates from her ageing frame. While her ears may not hear as well as a few years ago, she still likes to have them scratched by anyone who happens by. Rub her chest and you're her friend for life.

She sees me put on my joggers. The ears are alert and she waits for the next signal. I put on my favourite walking jacket. She is sitting at the front door. I pick up my keys and mobile phone. She is waiting for the lead to click to her collar. She looks out the door.

Our walks around the neighbourhood keep her senses alert and help to lessen the effects of canine senility, like barking at nothing in particular – especially at night. We have a ritual. I pick up the lead, she's panting, waiting for the door to open. We move outside and take a few steps. I drape the lead over her back while I collect the bags and scoop. I go back to her, pick up the lead and we set off. At each roadside, she stops and sits. I rub her chest and praise her. Along the way she plays the sniffing game. We walk down the street and suddenly she stops, almost wrenching my arm out of its socket. She draws the scent in deeply and sniffs around the area. She fully investigates every new blade of grass, tree and lightpost where an animal has paused and left a scent. Who has been here? Mmm, that's Ralph from down the street…we move a few more steps and pause again. It's easy to see who's the boss here. We reach the unleash area. She has a drink and wanders around, occasionally almost breaking into a trot. She loves meeting all the other dogs and their owners. There's always a person ready to give her a scratch.

It's a slow trek home playing the sniffing game until we reach the last, steep hill. She perks up at the two dogs that greet her through the gate at the top. They bark and attempt to break out. It inspires her to stand tall with ears erect and tail outstretched. She pulls on the lead and lets out a Woof! There's spark in the old girl yet! The three dogs jostle, and then it's over until next time. Seiko heads home. The tail drops and she is feeling her age again. For a moment, there was a flash of the pride and energy she had in her prime. Nearly home. She makes a few feeble attempts to sniff, but all she really wants is another drink and a long rest on her favourite bag.

Jenny Muller

Dummy spitting and tears

Dummy spits are okay sometimes. They help us remember that we're not just a cog in a hospital machine.

I had been brusquely sent into the CAT scan room to swallow the prep with hardly a word of explanation. It had been a big day, it was in the first months of my illness, I was tired, and, let's face it, angry for various reasons. As a nurse I knew what was happening, but it was not the moment for me to be a lamb. I rationalised that other people were being poorly treated if there was no information. So I REFUSED TO HAVE THE CAT SCAN! It was part of a research project and my not having it would delay the program timetable.

The research nurse was paged, I was 'counselled', I had a breather and a cup of tea and everything went ahead.

In the early months of diagnosis, I was very focused and organised. I had started chemo and bought a wig before my hair even fell out. I took it along on its stand to the Look Good…Feel Better session, keen to get the gift bag of cosmetics, have afternoon tea and chat with the other ladies. But I was running late and the only seat left was next to the demonstrator, which meant that I would be the model.

That was it – floodgates. No make-up would stay on my face. People were kind; I cried more. In the end, I just had to go home and settle down.

Tears well up when I haven't been able to process it all, a speechless overflow. But a good weep can enhance immune function the way laughter does. 'After the feeling comes the healing,' my support group says. A good cry is a good cry. With my wig in hand, I had pushed myself ahead of my feelings.

Later, I worked out the wig styling with the help of a friend. I booked in to another Look Good session, wore my wig and came away with my bag of make-up.

It's not always easy to remember, but I need to be gentle with myself. Sometimes there's a lot to get through.

A car full of roses

I zip off with my old friend Amy, in her raspberry-coloured car, to the Rose Society Summer Show. My husband smiles and waves us off at the gate. Yes, let's face it, he can do with a break from me. I have to laugh at Amy keeping up her subscription to the Society; it's pretty sedate, but she says it makes her feel like a spring chicken. And it's a good twenty years since we were that — hitting the town and having super fun.

It's not only that the flowers are gorgeous; I get a kick out of the suburban town hall with the neat signs, name-tagged rose officials, and the cardboard box on one of the official tables for the $2 admission. The display hall is loaded up with the perfume of competition blooms, the blue ribbons and honourable mentions. Amy introduces me to the society president, who must be flagging. He was up at four in the morning to arrange the enormous decorative bouquets and coordinate the judging. He's a big bloke, straightforward and apparently straight! Confident and patient enough to be straight, love roses, be good at flower arranging and being president.

In the refreshment room there are homemade sandwiches, cakes and slices, china cups and saucers and big metal tea pots. No polystyrene cups, dim sims or chips here. Anzac biscuits are for sale in cellophane bags. I buy a packet and slip them in Amy's bag when she goes to the loo.

I look in the mirror over the hand basin. I'm feeling pretty good. In the past it's been wheelchair, wig, wanting to throw up. But I've always come to the show, no matter what.

The show is winding up, the stalls being dismantled. On Amy's advice, we smile sweetly at the president and drive home with the backseat of the little raspberry car full of bunches of roses!

Self-absorbed? No way

I was walking on the treadmill at the rehab gym a couple of years after the secondaries showed up, recovering from being sick.

I complained to my physio that I was getting tired of being self-absorbed. I waited for him to say, 'Oh, no. You interact wonderfully with the other patients. You are so uncomplaining and positive.' Surely these things would be kind of true. But he didn't let me off the hook.

'It's a difficult thing to avoid,' he said, 'if you're dealing with a longstanding illness, especially being on a long course of painkillers.'

It has been hard, so I guess I can forgive myself when I forget to have fun and smell the roses.

Little fish

The little sucker fish, eighteen hours new from the shop, overnight became an ex-fish. In a word, dead.

My stepson came home yesterday with his first pet and a little fish tank, all that's manageable when you're renting. And now this. He rushed past looking as if he had killed it himself. He was off to the pet shop for the Tropical Fish Instruction Sheet, rather too late it seemed.

Sound from the kitchen. Son and dad are sorting out the funeral for the little fish. Chortling and chuckling. I've been sent out for saying, 'Goodbye, little fellow'. His interment has been downsized to being chucked in the kitchen bin with scraps and tea bags. They're onto the technical stuff – setting up the tank again.

My stepson was just a kid when I got sick seven years ago. His mum had breast cancer and she had died. So, I guess I panicked when I saw his face as he ran down the hall after his first pet death.

He's in there chuckling now, while his dad's voice bounces off the ceiling. They're having fun, and the little sucker fish will be fondly remembered.

Lesley Wilder

Chocolate frogs

My sofa

$\mathcal{M}$y favourite place to sit at home is in my family room, on my sofa. It is a recent purchase; a modern, yellow chaise longue. I have draped an animal print rug on it and scattered it with cushions. From there I can recline and look out on the lovely vista that is my garden.

Sunlight dapples through the trees and the contrast of leaves, rocks, grass and flowers fascinates me. The birds chatter as they socialise among the branches or take a bath in the terracotta saucers that top three posts placed in the garden.

My animals, two dogs and two cats, sit and watch – the dogs for an intruder on their territory – the cats, perhaps wondering if they can be fast enough, silent enough, to catch a bird. Yet the bells on their collars give our feathered friends the edge.

Jack, my three-year-old dog, is talking to me in his growling, yipping way through the gauze door, trying to cajole a pat or a feed, or both. My mind slips back in time to when he was a young puppy and allowed to come inside.

. . .

I am on my sofa, a different sofa – grey, and sagging in the middle where the supports have given way. Jack the puppy lies on my tummy, chewing my fingers, making them wet and warm with his breath.

'Ouch, Jack. Stop that!' I cry. He looks up at me cheekily with his little bat-like face. His eyes sparkle and his tongue lolls from his mouth as he pants happily. His company is dear to me. He helps me while away the time when I am too sick to go to work. My constant coughing doesn't offend him, and he has all the time in the world to wait while I breathlessly shuffle around.

Why won't my cough go away? I haven't been able to go to work for weeks. The doctors say it is asthma and prescribe inhalers. 'The coughing is causing the chest wall pain and the vomiting,' say the doctors. Weeks later when I can barely walk they tell me, 'The coughing has caused your lower back pain.'

My friends and family tentatively enquire, 'Is the cancer

back?' 'No,' I tell them. 'I've had x-rays and numerous blood tests but nothing shows up. They have even checked for Legionnaire's disease!'

. . .

My thoughts wander to months later. Clive and I sit in the surgeon's rooms. He studies the bone scan the GP ordered that finally rang alarm bells, and the CT scan that came afterwards. He has a student with him today and she sits unobtrusively in the background. Today's lesson – how to tell someone their cancer has metastasised. How to tell someone they are going to die.

But he does not impose a death sentence. He only says, 'Well my dear, we have a much harder battle on our hands this time. You should see the oncologist as soon as possible.'

Clive says, 'But we're going camping for Christmas.' The surgeon replies, 'The only camping you will be doing is at the hospital.' The student and I say nothing.

. . .

My reverie is broken by the noise of the mower starting up. My husband prepares to cut the grass and gather the clippings to mulch the garden. His loving care of the garden is matched by the loving care with which he tends me when I need him.

Children have come to play in the park just beyond our fence. Their laughter rings out and makes me smile. Life. It is all around me, not passing me by, but including me, lifting my spirits.

The wedding

he wedding day was hot and sticky, but the satin and lace of my dress felt cool and silky on my skin, rustling as I walked. I was the princess every little girl dreams of being on her wedding day. The quaint community hall was bordered by shimmering green cane fields. We nervously took our places before the celebrant. We stood under an archway made by Clive, entwined with ivy and decorated with two white bells.

* * *

The band played an Irish love song as Clive and I cut our wedding cake, our respective children, friends and relatives smiling and clapping, cheering us on.

If anything happened to you
If my worst fears ever came true
I'd have no reason to carry on through
If anything happened to you.

The hall and tables were decorated with flowers and candles in colours to match the bridesmaids' dresses: pink, mauve, peach, royal blue, jade and aubergine.

So promise me you will take care
It's a wicked old world out there
I'd be devastated, broken and blue
If anything happened to you.

On the dance floor, a dozen Irish dancers, including my three daughters, limbered up, preparing for their jigs and reels. The girls were beautifully made-up with their hair in masses of ribbons and curls, their dresses lavishly embroidered with Celtic designs, works of art fit to hang in a gallery. The boys looked handsome and statuesque in their kilts. The floor began to vibrate and the room came alive as the guests all clapped to the rhythm of the dancers' hard shoes and the strains of 'St Patrick's Day'. Then the girls were flying high, dancing a reel in their soft shoes, drawing gasps from the onlookers.

I heaved a sigh of relief. The event had been a huge success, and I felt a great sense of accomplishment to have reached that moment. You see, I had spent eight of the previous nine months undergoing chemotherapy and radiotherapy treatment for breast cancer.

. . .

The archway that we were married under now marks the entrance to our garden — a reminder of the vows we made that day.

Now we were nine

My family of three daughters aged seventeen, fourteen and ten now included a husband, his son aged nineteen and his three daughters aged sixteen, fifteen and eleven. Nine of us.

We had become The Brady Bunch.

Dragonfly

Five ladies sit in a small room. Two walls are taken up by crowded bookshelves, and two by windows closed against the noise of traffic from the busy intersection outside.

Two of those ladies are professionals; one is a social worker, the other a psychologist. There is a device on the coffee table in the centre of the group from which, with the aid of Telstra, come the voices of two other ladies. One is not well enough to travel and the other lives in another town. That's seven ladies altogether. They all have a bond and that bond is advanced breast cancer.

The purpose of the group meeting, for one hour each week, is to discuss the day-to-day experiences of living with this stage of the disease; to discuss various treatments, doctors, family and financial concerns and, on occasion, our fears of dying.

Kerry, a group member who lived in a rural area west of Brisbane, was always able to fill any awkward silences with interesting tidbits about her life. Like the time she and her husband won a weekend for two on the Gold Coast. Yes, we heard some juicy details.

Early on, Kerry told us of her ex-fiancé who had died of cancer. At his funeral a white dove was released. A white feather floated down from the flying dove and landed on Kerry's breast. The following week she learned that she had cancer in that breast.

She told us she believed in animal 'signs'. She said that the three dragonflies she had watched that morning buzzing at her kitchen window signified change coming.

One of the ladies listening in the room thought that this was all just a bit too fanciful for her, until the following day when she was presented with a gift for being a guest speaker at an unrelated breast cancer function. The gift was a dragonfly brooch.

Kerry inspired us for months with stories of her and her husband's struggle to raise money to fit out a bus so that she could experience her dream of travelling around Australia before she died. Many people helped, notably her local member of parliament and the entrepreneur, Dick Smith.

Several of us travelled to an open day at Kerry and Brian's home, aptly named Dragon's Hollow. The walls of their lounge room were adorned with photos of their mediaeval-style wedding and certificates attesting to courses they had taken in mediaeval arts. We inspected the refit of the bus they had acquired through a local bus company. Brian had done all the work with some assistance from Kerry, and they were both very proud.

We then enjoyed a sausage sizzle as Kerry and Brian cut a cake decorated with a bus on an open road, and we wished them bon voyage. The local paper ran the story and included a photo of the neighbours, friends, family and local MP all grouped in front of the bus which was emblazoned with the name 'Dragon's Express'. A south-east Queensland television program also took up the story. Kerry was no shrinking violet and obviously enjoyed the attention.

During our weekly sessions, Kerry phoned in to give us a glimpse of where they were and where they had been. She told us of her difficulties obtaining her prescription painkiller interstate and we pondered ways to get around this problem. It was probably the same for other people, we thought. This could be an issue that needs action.

Unfortunately, the trip was much shorter than Kerry and Brian had hoped. Kerry has since taken another journey to a place where she can't phone us. She does send messages though.

The lady who had earlier been presented with the dragonfly brooch was travelling to Kerry's funeral, running late and stressing that she was not on the right road. As she waited at the lights of an intersection, a car towing a boat pulled alongside. Being a bit of a boatie she looked it over. The name on the bow? 'Dragonfly'. 'All right Kerry', she laughed. 'I'll calm down. This must be the right way!'

I have since seen a Kevin Costner movie that tells of a woman desperately trying to send a message to her husband from 'beyond'. The name of the movie? You guessed it. *Dragonfly*.

Fighting spirit

*I*t was late evening, and as is my habit, I was watching television and crocheting while I waited for Clive to finish his shift. We have a taxi business and he drives one of the taxis from three in the afternoon until three in the morning.

Only my youngest stepdaughter and daughter now live with us, and they come and go at odd times.

My stepdaughter Rebecca arrived home from visiting a former school friend's mother who was very ill with cancer. Instead of just muttering, 'Hello, I'm tired, I'm going to bed,' and heading for her room, she surprised me from behind with a big hug. 'Thanks for having such a fighting spirit,' she said.

I felt touched. Perhaps there is still hope for us to become close…

Karaoke

I was sitting at Day Oncology in the public hospital waiting for treatment, enjoying the CD that was playing. It sounded like an Irish ballad singer. Yes.

Oh Danny Boy, Oh Danny Boy, I love you so...

A bit different to the usual modern music the younger nurses like to put on. The nurse attending to me said, 'We have live music today.' I thought she was referring to the patients singing along in the next room. People were even clapping.

I continued with my writing project, listening to the classic songs being sung. The music seemed louder, closer — were they changing the speakers around?

'And now, for you Neil Diamond lovers...'

'Hands touching hands, reaching out, touching me, touching you... Sweet Caroline.'

I looked up and there was this bald guy, in pyjamas and slippers with a hospital name tag on his wrist, singing into a karaoke machine!

I fought back tears listening to his beautiful voice, the joy shared by his fellow patients.

Resting

The water dragon lies stretched out along half the length of the fish pond, basking in the sun. The fish swim around him, nonplussed, the sun flashing on their silver or golden bodies as they suck on the mossy stones or splash under the waterfall. The sound of running water is mesmerising, calming and peaceful.

Today I am resting, gathering my thoughts and strength after a big week.

My eldest daughter lost her baby. The baby, though unplanned and barely formed, had already found a place in our hearts and our lives. The scans showed us its presence, and the doctor's report recorded its heartbeat. But it wasn't to be. In the cold atmosphere of hospital casualty I put my arms around Katherine and said 'Life's tough, ain't it?' Katherine replied, 'I'm tough too, Mum.' I wondered, then, whether I have been too outwardly brave in the past. Perhaps it would be better to let others glimpse my vulnerability.

The week ended with Zoe's graduation. Our feelings of sadness over Katherine and Murray's loss were mixed with pride and happiness for Zoe's achievement, the beginning of a new chapter in her life.

Tonight we celebrate the engagement of Anthony and Vanna, who are beginning a new chapter in their lives too.

Two years ago I would not have believed I would be here to experience these milestones, and because of that, I savour them all the more.

Hair raisers

*I*t was Christmas Day and my mother, sister, niece and nephew had joined us for lunch.

As I served the food, my eighteen-year-old nephew said, 'Aunty Les, now you're having chemo, will you lose your hair?'

'Yes Ben. I have lost my hair already.'

He looked at me puzzled, so I lifted my wig and he gasped. My wig looked so much like my usual hairstyle he had not twigged!

Support groupie

'Oh you're just a groupie!' Veronica joked.

The six of us at the table had a chuckle as we sipped cups of tea or coffee. I had that afternoon mentioned, in various conversations, three different people I knew from other support groups I belonged to.

One group is for people with all types of cancer; the second is for people with breast cancer, and I say 'people' because the group includes two males with breast cancer; the third is for women with advanced breast cancer.

Those of us sitting at the 'Coffee Club' were part of the third group.

In the advanced breast cancer group, we have an hour-long weekly session with a social worker and a psychologist. Now it has spilled over to a regular gathering afterwards for a coffee and general chat. This in turn has led to more social events: a dinner party, a few barbecues, shopping expeditions, four-wheel driving and a trip to Sydney. We have found that although our husbands may be reluctant to join a support group, they feel quite comfortable having a natter around a barbecue.

Though based in Brisbane, this group is open to women throughout Queensland by means of teleconferencing. They may be unable to attend the group in person due to failing health, treatment, doctor's appointments, or even travelling. The number of those attending in person and those phoning in has fluctuated since late 2001, and can be anywhere from three to a dozen.

A couple of the out-of-town 'phone-in' ladies have, on occasion, travelled to Brisbane for treatment and been able to visit in person. This strengthens the bond that has already grown from the weekly telephone discussions.

I joined the group for people with all types of cancer in April 2001. It was my first experience of a support group other than Nursing Mothers, which I joined in desperation when my third daughter was six months old. The local paper said that the Quality of Life Support Group (Southside branch) was being formed and would be meeting twice a month at the church three doors away from my house. How could I not join in?

The other members are mostly older but very caring people, and a few of them have since become like extended family to me. As most are dealing with different cancers, and are at different stages, I empathise but do not compare myself with these people.

I tried a local group for women with breast cancer, but it was mainly comprised of women with primary cancers. There was only one other woman who had secondaries and those were in her bones. I was having treatment for liver, lung and bone secondaries and was quite weak at that time. I was treated like an invalid, which I guess I was. It is a bit scary to be the one with the worst prognosis. They didn't quite know what to say to me and I wasn't sure how much they wanted me to say to them.

It was shortly after this that I found the group for women with advanced breast cancer. I knew it was just what I was looking for, where I belonged. Unable to maintain my full-time career, I had been lost and lonely. I had to find new interests that didn't cost money as our finances had become strained with the loss of my income. I had to find new friends to spend time with during the week, as most of my old friends worked. I seemed to 'click' with the girls who attended this group. When my husband met them he felt comfortable with them and their partners too. I began to feel normal again.

Discussion within the group made me realise I was eligible to claim my superannuation benefits as well as total and permanent disability insurance. The money has alleviated some of our financial difficulties and others in the group have also since benefited from successful insurance claims.

I had heard good things about a breast cancer support group in a nearby bayside area. When my husband's aunt was diagnosed with breast cancer and wanted to join a support group, I suggested we go along to this bayside group. I have since attended three meetings and a funeral with them and although I only meant to ease my aunt into the group, I think I may keep going.

This group is mainly comprised of people with primary cancers, but I have changed since my earlier experience. My health has become stronger and my confidence has grown. I don't think I scare people any more. I am a reminder that cancer can come back later than the 'magic five-year goal'. I am a reminder that people need to stay attuned to their bodies.

The hospital occupational therapist came to visit me one day when I was having treatment. I had casually admitted to the oncology nurse that I was a bit down. This particular nurse was very attuned to me. That was all I had to say and the right professional was there to give advice. I was grieving for several of my support group friends. One had decided to stop treatment and death was imminent. One had lost the use of her limbs and was confined to a wheelchair. Another, who had so recently seemed to exude life and energy, had had a relapse and was very ill in hospital.

The OT said, 'Well, unfortunately this is the trouble with support groups. Inevitably you are going to see people's heath decline, and some will die. You can't help but identify with that and become depressed.'

I immediately went into defence mode, something my husband knows all about!

'I am not depressed,' I sniffed into a tissue. 'I am just grieving for my friends; for the loss they are experiencing, whether it is the use of their limbs, their energy or possibly their life. Isn't that natural? Each one is an amazing woman and I feel privileged to have had the opportunity of meeting and knowing them all.'

Of those three women, one is making a recovery, one is stable and one has passed on. I was the spokesperson for two support groups at the funeral of the woman who died. I was very nervous but not upset. I had done my grieving when she had decided to stop treatment. She knew her time had come. Her funeral was, in fact, uplifting; a celebration of the life of an amazing woman.

Some of my family think I am dwelling on my disease. They prefer to pretend it's not really happening. For me, it is a reality I have learned to live with by getting involved with it. My way, I guess, of feeling some sort of control. I believe this has been made possible by giving and receiving the support of others who are riding the same emotional roller-coaster that is life with cancer.

The envelope

I said I would wait in the car while Clive went into Kentucky Fried Chicken to buy takeaway – neither of us felt like cooking dinner after the day we'd had.

On my lap was the CT scan, the first since diagnosis eight years ago. I was desperate to read the report, though Clive wanted me to wait to see the doctor tomorrow.

I held the envelope, checking Clive's progress in the queue to the counter.

I carefully opened the packet and slid out the report. It read '…pulmonary (lung) metastases, pathological rib fractures, extensive hepatic (liver) metastatic disease and malignant bony infiltration and destruction of the sacrum and left ileum…'

I'm going to die!

Clive was paying for the chicken. My heart pounding, I quickly returned the report to its envelope and placed it on the floor of the car. Clive was walking back to the car. I took a deep breath and smiled at him as he got closer.

Two years and five months have passed since that day. I have since enjoyed the weddings of two stepdaughters, held two newborn step-grandchildren and attended my youngest daughter's graduation. I have been inspired by the many new acquaintances in my widened social scene. My journey with cancer has been made easier through the efforts of those who have gone before me. Because of this, I would like to help make things easier for those who follow.

Yes, I'm going to die, but not quite yet.

Anne Pennington

Chocolate frogs

Not afraid of dying

My GP has a student with him. We're chatting. It's a routine visit.

I have no tension, no anxiety.

'You're not afraid of dying, are you?' He asks me matter-of-factly.

I'm taken aback. I've never thought about it before.

Is it because I'm not afraid of dying that I have broken my journey with breast cancer into small components and dealt with them, each one, a step, one step at a time? 'Bridges' I call them.

Is it because I'm not afraid of dying that I'm able to see the many things that make up who I am? That the cancer is just one of them?

Is it because I'm not afraid of dying that I'm able to enjoy the sand between my toes as the waves crash in, a joke, a giggle, and a jolly good laugh?

Is it because I'm not afraid of dying that I savour the crisp fresh air of a new day, out with friends or at work, and the smell of coffee bubbling up on the stove?

Is it because I am not in continual pain, that I have no nausea? That it's not in my organs yet? That I'm not physically affected in any way? Is that why I'm not afraid of dying?

Morning walk

First light
turns the black of night
away
this crisp October morning.

Today I don't see
the beauty, the freshness of it all.
You see – last evening
I was told I have breast cancer.

One foot steps
then the other
as I walk the track
around the lake
without any conscious thought,
striving for order
as I find myself
on my routine walk.

I'm on my own
with only
the ducks, waterhen
and graceful old swan,
busy
finding food
preening
saying, hello day.

They don't notice me.
They don't notice the tears
sliding quietly down my face.
They don't ask questions.

Who'll look after my treasures
when I'm gone?
Notes people have written me,
press clippings and mementos,
The stuff in the top drawers
of my desk and dresser.

Fi can have the ice-cream maker,
The one I've never used.
She'll make use of it.
Vanessa said years ago
she'd like my dinner set.
Should I give it to someone closer?

I'm on the other side of the lake now.
My thoughts wander to
What happens now?
What happens next?
When will I find out?

Ceri will know.
She'll answer my questions.

The ducks, waterhen
and graceful old swan
don't notice
that my tears
have subsided.

The long lunch

Silver cutlery, tall elegant wine glasses and fine linen napkins are set precisely on the crisp white tablecloths which stretch forever on the gnarled old wood of the wharf.

The sun shines brilliantly while a gentle breeze cools the air.

The river stretches away, bordered by graceful old red gums. The brown water lazily makes its way on its long journey to the river mouth. Boats float gently and people bask in the sunshine, making the most of their late summer holidays.

On the wharf, champagne and other fine wines flow freely. The hubbub of chatter is interrupted as Rosie whoops with laughter at Adrian's joke. We all join in, getting noisier as the mood takes us over.

We pass plates of luscious food up and down the table – the dark red of the smoked venison contrasts with the soft pink of the trout. Lorraine's long red-tipped fingers elegantly reach for a pink-ripe fig wrapped in prosciutto.

When the chef lifts the lid, we all turn to gasp at the sight of the Murray cod lined up on the barbecue. Jenny reaches for her camera to capture the image forever.

Judy and Gary join in with the quartet now singing at the other end of the table.

And we're stayin' alive, stayin' alive

Ah, ha, ha, ha, stayin' alive

We all join in, marking the rhythm by clicking our fingers and clinking our spoons, while the paddle steamer gives a steam boosted toot.

I bask in the beauty of the surroundings, the company of friends not seen for a long while, and the food and wine.

It was not so long ago that things were different...

Chemo the second time around

The staff still know when to joke and when silence is best, and how to conquer the most stubborn veins. The poles still look like TV antennae attached to each chair in the circle.

The coffee machine in the kitchen is new; it looks as if I will need a licence to drive it. Another time. I make myself a cup of tea and head back into the room to find a chair – just as I did last time round.

I sit and wait my turn. And then it hits me – I'm alone. I have to get through this on my own this time.

Jenny was with me before. We met when we had adjoining rooms in hospital. We were having surgery on the same day, we shared the same surgeon and the same oncologist, and later we had chemotherapy treatments together. We compared notes on the highs and the lows, while our friendship grew to coffees and special occasions.

Over coffee she told me of party plans to celebrate her daughter's engagement. A marquee would be set up in her glorious garden, surrounded by creamy magnolias, camellias and azaleas. Lights would shine on the tree trunks – the silver of the birches, the shiny smoothness of the crepe myrtles. Guests would arrive through a canopy festooned with flowers.

But Jenny is not with me this time – she's well, thank goodness. I am alone; the tears slide quietly down my face as I wonder if I can cross this bridge without her.

Total information pack

I have been hungry for information ever since I was diagnosed with breast cancer. In the early days, I found the National Breast Cancer Centre's booklet *All About Early Breast Cancer* and *Dr Susan Love's Breast Book* the most useful. When you could find it, there was an impressive amount of written material covering the medical aspects of breast cancer.

Later, I realised that important – not necessarily medical – information was available. It was given by other women, friends and breast cancer compatriots. I found out about things such as the Victorian Patient Transport Assistance Scheme, which subsidises transport and accommodation for patients having to travel more than one hundred kilometres for treatment, the Medicare Safety Net, the Pharmaceutical Benefits Scheme Safety Net, and the fact that the Lymphoedema Clinic in Melbourne runs two-day education sessions for those diagnosed with, or at risk of, lymphoedema. I did not find out from medical practitioners or hospital services.

My former work colleague and friend, Jan, died recently. Jan's bowel cancer had spread to her liver by the time she was diagnosed. One day our treatments coincided. She was in the oncology ward for chemotherapy treatment. I was there for Aredia, a monthly bisphosphonate treatment for my bones.

'They should give you a total information pack,' she said as she lay back on the recliner chair. 'One that gives you all you need to know, that includes all the financial info as well as the other stuff.'

I still can't believe Jan is no longer with us. I remember the 'staff meetings' over a glass or two of champagne, her ribbing me about the endless lists that I make, or rocking back and forth when I am deep in thought. I remember the last time I saw her. 'I'll see you again soon,' she said to me. I left the hospital with tears in my eyes, knowing that it would not be possible.

I'll find a way for us to get 'Total Information Packs'. And I'll dedicate them to Jan.

Only half the story

*I*t's only half the story,' I think after the presentation by the Director at a Cancer Council seminar. For the last half hour he had used a computer-generated display of facts and figures about different types of cancers and the numbers of people affected. His figures were from the Cancer Registry.

As the Registry's pamphlet says, this information is used, among other things, to:

Help in planning for and improving services to care for cancer patients

Measure the quality and effectiveness of cancer treatments

Provide data for research

Help with studies to find out what causes cancer.

Although it is currently a legal requirement to report diagnosis of initial disease, there is no such requirement to report advanced disease.

As the Director is speaking I wonder, 'How will they be able to plan for and improve services to care for patients with advanced disease if they don't know that I, and many others like me, *have* advanced disease?'

The issue is brought home to me that night when I arrive home and open my mail. 'I am writing to you because the Cancer Registry has been notified that you have been diagnosed with breast cancer…I would like to ask you to take part in a national research study…' the Director of the Cancer Registry writes.

'I'll never be randomly selected like this for a research study into advanced breast cancer,' I think as I read his letter.

'How can governments plan, how can medical services be improved, how can the right samples be selected for the right research studies? How can the Director of the Cancer Council tell the whole story if no one knows how many people are living with advanced cancer?' I ask myself.

I have heard excuses such as 'It's too costly', 'What about privacy laws?' and 'Doctors and hospitals won't do it because it is too time consuming and too difficult'. Probably the same excuses that were put forward before the law was passed requiring reporting of initial disease. A way round was found then, why not now?

I have advanced disease. It matters to me that I receive the best and most effective treatment and care. To be the best, such treatment and care must be informed by current data and knowledge. I want the whole story.

But the story will not be complete until it is mandatory to report diagnosis of spread of disease.

The good things

Luck, good fortune, a silver lining, call it what you will. I have experienced it all since my diagnosis with breast cancer.

Like the day I received an email from the Breast Cancer Network Australia asking if I would be interested in participating in a writing project for women with advanced breast cancer. 'Inspirational Women' they called it.

'I'm not inspirational, and I can't write,' I thought. At the same time, I was chuffed that I had been asked.

'The work will be guided, revised and edited by professional writer, Christine Gillespie', the project guidelines stated. I had participated in a writing workshop connected with the Warrior Women project with Christine before. I knew what a cathartic experience it was, even if I didn't feel confident as a writer afterwards!

I would give it a go.

I have travelled so far since the day that I went for my mammogram that time, referred by my GP. I lay on the ultrasound table just prior to my diagnosis. I was not overly concerned or anxious as I had a history of benign breast lumps. In fact, I was impressed with their thoroughness as they performed a fine needle biopsy. Even when the nurse held my hand as the radiologist undertook the procedure I thought, 'How kind and caring!'

Not long afterwards, I lay on the trolley all prepped and ready for theatre — a bilateral mastectomy as a result of having tumours in both breasts, two infiltrating lobular carcinomas in my right breast and an infiltrating ductal carcinoma in my left breast. It felt as if I was in a bay in a milking shed. The man in the next bay began describing the surgery he was about to undergo to his lungs for what was clearly metastatic disease. 'Too much information,' I thought, but I also remember thinking how fortunate I was by comparison.

My boss has been unending in his support since my diagnosis, having me undertake work at a level of responsibility that matched my health at any given point. He has allowed me to work flexibly, adjusting my hours according to how well I feel and to keep medical appointments. His support, plus that of my colleagues, has been immeasurable.

I have met many amazing women. Out of the blue I received a phone call from Raelene Boyle who is active in breast cancer advocacy. She took the time and trouble to ring me shortly after my diagnosis 'to tell it to me straight'. The women who are active in advocacy and support are generous with their time and expertise, and all work tirelessly to ensure better experiences and outcomes for women with breast cancer.

I have had the opportunity to undertake training and, with support and mentoring, have gone on to participate in some breast cancer advocacy work myself. I find this work challenging and rewarding, and I have met wonderful people.

Jenny, whom I met while in hospital, has become a special friend through our support of each other through surgery, chemotherapy, and the time that followed.

I have experienced wonderful care, support and love from my husband, friends, family and work colleagues. They seem to know what to say and do at any given point. Many remarked how my hospital room resembled a florist shop with boxes, bouquets, and posies of flowers covering every available surface.

None of this would have occurred if I had not been diagnosed with breast cancer.

This writing project has been wonderful, enjoyable and agonising. Christine's ideas, suggestions, and gentle editing, all by teleconference and email, have been an immense support.

I hope the reader will find, as I have, the material in this collection as well as the beautiful way it has been written, truly inspirational.

Monique Skarke

Climbing the walls

A catering woman entered my room apologetically to retrieve my breakfast tray. I remained perched on the edge of the hospital bed, hesitant to move an inch for fear of more sharp pains shooting through my torso and left arm. I smiled at the kitchen lady and said, 'Thank you.' What I really wanted to do was let out the primal scream of a mortally wounded caveman.

The hunched-up shoulders of an octogenarian with osteoporosis had replaced my youthful posture of the previous day. In one day, I had lost fifteen lymph nodes from under my left arm and fifty years of energy. I felt like a wet sponge. To save my life from a malignant cancer, all my verve must be taken away through the constant pain of surgery, chemotherapy and radiotherapy. Now I could be at least eighty-five per cent certain that my cancerous breast lump, removed with two cancerous lymph nodes, would not kill my body. But my flesh, bones, and psyche had become dead to me.

An alien in a foreign land, I waited for the physiotherapist. The other women arriving for pre-op admission were all much older than me, but many had the same diagnosis; breast cancer.

'Hey, I'm young and healthy!' I wanted to tell everyone who passed by my open door. 'It's all a BIG mistake. Could you put me back together again like I was before? Please? And for God's sake get this bloody parasite of a wound drain out of my body so I can dress myself and shower normally!'

A woman with military posture and zeal entered my hospital room. The embroidered buttons on her crisply ironed blouse were of another era. In a prim, authoritarian manner this health commando told me that she was the physiotherapist assigned to show me the post-operative rehabilitation exercises.

I was keen to get on with it so that this straight-laced creature who looked like she was straight from a bible study seminar would leave me alone to sulk, with my trashy magazines to comfort me.

In the harried manner of a stressed person, the physiotherapist handed me a poor quality photocopy. The sickly green-coloured paper contained a list of exercises for me. I examined the finely stitched embroidery on the centre panel of the crisp white blouse as she gave me a stream of prim, authoritarian instructions.

My left arm hung limply by my side. I wished it was invisible. Then the torture began.

'Please lift your left arm as high as you can.'

I grunted, guttural sounds of pain.

'Can you lift it any higher? I know it hurts, but you need to get it moving or you will get a *frozen shoulder.*'

I've never met anyone with a frozen shoulder, but it didn't sound very good, so I persevered. Despite my intense pain and obvious commitment to lifting my arm as ordered, there was no response from the commando. Good girl. Well done. Yes! No! Nothing. Wasn't positive reinforcement supposed to bring good results in students? She frowned at my limp arm as I raised it with greater effort towards the heavens.

I felt as if I was being judged. Would I fail this rehabilitation test?

With a supreme effort I lifted my arm a few more centimetres from the left side of my body. The movement caused the most intense pain of my life, even greater than childbirth! It was as though a sadistic attacker was ripping my arm off. All this to please the physiotherapist!

'Now come over here and stand next to the wall. I want you to walk your fingers up the wall – slowly – like this.'

I watched as the pain seared through my arm and reached my fingertips. The physio demonstrated, with authoritative fingers, walking up the walls.

Great, now they want me to literally climb the walls. That's what I've been doing mentally since I got here!

I tried to copy the exercise. 'Good, just a bit higher,' she said. 'I want you to lower your arm again and repeat this exercise six times, twice a day.'

God, I'll be lucky to survive two of these torture sessions a day! How much pain does this woman think I can endure? I wondered if my face was revealing my agony. I didn't want to appear weak, so I had tried to hide my pain for the sake of my personal dignity as a strong, fit, young woman. Yeah, a strong, fit, young woman with malignant breast cancer who can't lift her left arm above her shoulder.

'That should do it for today. I'll be back on Tuesday to run through some more exercises with you. Make sure that you take some pain relief at least half an hour before these exercise sessions next time.'

'OK,' I reply lamely. What I really want to say is: If I'd known you were coming to torture me I would have had some pethidine in preparation!

I want to hate her, but she is only doing her job, so I decide to try and be friendlier next time we meet. Even when I have been tortured, I want to please my torturer and not upset her by complaining about the lack of warning to take painkillers before the session.

I politely say goodbye and collapse onto the firm hospital bed. Oh to curl up in a foetal ball and roll off the edge of the earth…I want to disappear from my life, to no longer exist – not in this condition anyway.

At last my lunch arrives and I can begin eating again – the most enjoyable way to pass the time in hospital. After three very boring and pain-filled days my clothes are already starting to pinch around the waist and thighs. Never mind, a girl's gotta have some enjoyment in life!

Later that afternoon I request some pain medication to prepare for another torture session. Because I am doing the exercises alone this time, my mind is focused on more than how pissed off I am with the physio for making me do such painful exercises. I close my eyes and imagine that I am standing on the edge of a glacier on Mt Everest, reaching up for an icy overhang…

Really, I am standing in a weird position in my bland hospital room with my left arm stretched out, my fingers walking like a disabled spider up the wall. I grimace. I will probably never climb Mt Everest now. Tears begin to well up. I always wanted to trek to base camp, and maybe even climb higher. All of these adventures were still possible when I was young and healthy. Now my world is smaller and limited by the physical disabilities that cancer has brought with it.

Fed up with the exercises, I grab a chocolate bar from my top drawer and plonk myself on the bed. Supported by several pillows, I distractedly flick through one of my trashy magazines – slowly I begin to relax.

Luxury spa

The chemotherapy nurses had friendly faces but the room was cold, clinical and claustrophobic. No windows. No view at all. How could I spend several hours every week here? Every Monday, for the rest of my life.

Before, at the Mercy Private, I could see the Melbourne CBD, Fitzroy Gardens, South Melbourne and the water of Port Phillip Bay beyond. This new place was a complete downer, worse than I'd imagined. I doubted my decision to come here for my weekly treatments.

Should I go back to the Mercy despite the inconvenience? Despite the memories of pain and loss that the Mercy holds for me? Confusion fogged my brain as I continued to smile and chat with a nurse called Andrea.

Clichés are a handy way for the brain to focus on a thought that can lead to a decision: Maybe a change is as good as a holiday?

Yes, that's it! My regular Monday chemotherapy treatments will be MY DAY. Like a beauty session at a flash, expensive day spa. But without the luxury and the beauty treatments. Yes! I will still have the pampering (the Jason Recliner); IV hydration (water is great for the skin); and I could sit undisturbed. No whining toddler or poo-filled nappies while I read glossy magazines all afternoon. WOW…chemo! What a buzz! To my impressionable, drug-numbed brain the chemo experience was becoming more attractive by the second.

Julie Pallot

Worth the walk

One small window overlooked a T-intersection. The visitors all said they had a lovely view down to St Patrick's Cathedral. It was wasted on me though. I could not see outside from the bed. However, the window showed me day turning to night and back to day again. The hospital room was a small cubicle. Framed, nondescript prints on the white walls tried to add some interest. The hospital bed, lots of chrome and pillows piled high, allowed me to recline comfortably.

At the other end of the room was the door to the outside world. Nurses, doctors and visitors came and went, but it was an unknown to me. I could just catch glimpses of movement up and down the corridor. When would I see what was beyond this room?

I was connected to many drips, some with painkillers and others with medication to ward off infections. Blue plastic cylinders were wrapped around each leg, like the blue li-lo that I used to lounge on in the pool, lapping up the coolness of the water on a hot summer day. These leg wrappings did the opposite. They made me so hot. The motor pumped air into them. They inflated. The motor turned off. They deflated. I had these attached twenty-four hours a day and slept with the click of the motor going on and off every couple of minutes. The blue li-loes, pumping up and going flat, were to stop blood clots.

I had been in bed for five days. The surgeon had removed a large tumour from my leg. This could only be done by replacing my hip, removing half of my femur bone and having a large metal rod inserted.

The physiotherapist and two nurses came into the room to help me stand up for the first time. Would I be able to do it? How much of a limp would I have? The li-loes were disconnected. The motor went silent; peace at last! My heart beat loudly as they encouraged me to sit up on the edge of the bed with the nurses supporting my leg. On went my slippers and dressing gown. 'Now lean on me and let me take your weight,' said the physiotherapist.

Are you mad? Of course I would. I wasn't going to rush into this! What about the pain? What if my leg couldn't take the weight? I slowly put my feet onto the floor and slid further towards the edge of the bed. I took a deep breath and stood up. My head spun and I felt the pulse in my neck quicken. My hands were all clammy. I stood still for what seemed hours. It was really just a few seconds before a walking frame was placed in front of me. Tears came to my eyes. I'm not an old lady yet, I thought. I slowly took my own weight with the aid of the frame.

'Now, we are going to try to take some steps,' directed the physiotherapist. 'You move the frame forward first and then take a step with your good leg.' I followed her directions. 'Now do the same but step forward with your "bed" leg.' Again I followed her directions.

I did it! I can walk, I'm not a cripple. I took a few more steps and I was at the door. The staff sitting at the nurses' station cheered for me. I peered out into the unknown world beyond.

I turned around and walked back towards the side of the bed. Tentatively I detoured and stopped at the window to look out at my visitors' view. The roads were wet with early spring rain that freshened everything. New leaves were appearing on the large deciduous trees and the roads were congested with peak-hour traffic. People heading for the tram stop concentrated on their own thoughts, oblivious to being observed from my window. I could see the spire of St Patrick's Cathedral, a place I had visited often. A serene place, surrounded by gardens filled with early spring flowers. How very special the view was at this moment. Well worth the hard work of walking.

The cafe

I could smell freshly ground coffee as we opened the door of the cafe. We moved quietly among the small tables. We ordered coffee and a sandwich and sat next to the window. I was with my ex-husband. He had accompanied me to the first appointment with my medical oncologist. I had been diagnosed the previous week with advanced breast cancer, and had not been able to think, eat or sleep since. There were so many unanswered questions.

The oncologist's rooms had green leather seats. Everything was neat and orderly with a degree of opulence I had never seen in a doctor's rooms before. His back faced the window overlooking the tree tops in Victoria Parade. He was a lean man who reminded me of my father; quietly spoken, a gentleman in full control. I could not take in everything that was discussed, but a few things stayed in my mind.

'You have advanced breast cancer,' he said. 'The cancer has spread to the bone. Unfortunately, advanced breast cancer is not curable.'

The oncologist was saying what everyone else had avoided.

'The prognosis at the moment is not life-threatening and there are various treatments available,' he continued. 'I would suggest having your ovaries radiated and radiation treatment on the sternum where the bone secondary is.'

'How do I live with this prognosis?'

'Put your affairs in order,' he said. 'Then forget all about it and live your life to the full.'

I thanked the doctor for his truthfulness and decided to proceed with the treatments he suggested.

In the cafe, I looked out the window at the trams rattling past and at the people hurrying by under the protection of umbrellas, struggling to keep them under control in the strong wind. The coffee arrived and my thoughts started to come together.

My ex-husband sat opposite me and finally broke the silence

between us. 'You must be quite happy with what the doctor had to say,' he said.

'What do you mean, happy!'

'Well, he didn't say you were going to die now.'

'No I'm not going to die now. But I have to face a life-threatening illness. I have to live with this every day. And early menopause. Do you understand?' My voice sounded feeble.

His eyes lifted as if he was looking up for guidance, but I could see that he was unable or unwilling to understand what I was trying to tell him.

'I have been in the depths of depression since you left us,' I said. 'I've battled to get back on top of everything. I may have to face depression again as part of menopause. I'm frightened. I don't want to go back to where I was before.' I was so angry.

'I think you are over-reacting. Yes you may be going to die, but not now.'

'I can't believe we were both at the same appointment. We've come away with completely different facts,' I said.

He had his own agenda. Everything had to be all right.

He had been having an affair. When I found out, he packed his bags and moved in with the woman. No concern for the girls or for me. 'I love her,' he told me. 'You'll be okay.'

I don't know which was worse; having breast cancer or having the person I loved most in the world turn his back on me and leave me to pick up the pieces. To deal with not just my own hurt, but with that of our three beautiful daughters.

This latest development was not fitting in with his plans.

No, he was not there for me. I needed to take control of my own destiny, to gather together my own strength to fight this disease. It was the beginning of my journey; I was not giving up. I wanted to be around for as long as possible, but with no false expectations either. My three daughters, who I love dearly, were relying on me to fight and fight hard. To move on with my life. The last thing I needed was to be held back by someone who could not face the truth.

It's a while since I sat in that cafe for the first time. It has become a part of my life. After my treatments at this hospital, I have coffee there. I'm a stronger and happier person now than the frightened and lost lady who sat in that cafe eight years ago.

A weekend with Bev

The curtains let in a small ray of early morning light. In the bed lay a pale, fragile figure almost swallowed up by the pillows. The bed clothes were pulled up under her chin with the covers neat, smooth and lifeless.

The body in the bed came to life with a smile for her two visitors. The wig was missing and she wore no make-up. Unusual. The smile allowed me to regain my composure and give my good friend Bev a big hug. Bev had recently been given the news that all advanced breast cancer patients dread. She had only a few weeks to live. My daughter Kate and I had travelled to Adelaide to visit her.

Tony, Bev's husband, helped her out of bed and she joined us in the family room. The television was on but I cannot remember what shows we watched. The television was a comfort. It helped in the moments of silence and when Bev fell asleep. We watched a video of the time we met on a tour of America. We were both battling advanced breast cancer and something drew us together, a mutual understanding and the beginnings of a close friendship that could not be explained to others.

Bev's son, my daughter, Tony, Bev and I spent the weekend in the family room surrounded by family photos. From there we could see Bev's special rose garden that she had recently finished. The beautiful pale pink 'Seduction' rose was in plentiful bloom, as if it had been ordered to flower earlier than normal just for Bev. We talked, held hands and laughed over stories and memories while Tony fed us, made cups of tea and lovingly administered medication to Bev.

Bev kept falling asleep but would not go back to bed other than to sleep at night. The next morning, she demanded that Tony get her up so we could sit in the family room again and continue where we had left off. Not one moment was allowed to be wasted.

It was finally time to go back to the airport. What to say? How to say it? I looked at her and said I would visit again next month. This was just a game; we both knew this would be the last time I would see her. We hugged, holding back the tears. Bev went to hospital two days after we left and never came home again. My other daughter, Nicole, sang at Bev's funeral and I was a pall-bearer. As an advanced breast cancer sufferer, I could have floundered, but I seemed to gain the strength to face this loss. Bev's gift to me is the will to fight as hard as I can, just as she had.

Bev's husband gave me a gift recently; two pale pink 'Seduction' roses. I have made a rose garden which I can see from my family room. Julie's rose garden dedicated to her dear friend Bev.

The unit

he door to the oncology unit is straight opposite my oncologist's waiting rooms. I had been attending these rooms for a couple of years before I finally got to see what was behind this door. I had no desire to investigate. It was an unknown world which I was quite happy to leave unknown.

The unit holds no mysteries any more. I have been visiting every four weeks for five years. Sixty-four treatments, reclining in comfortable blue chairs where you can put your feet up. Each chair has a pole attached for the intravenous bag. The chairs are set in a circle so that all the patients can see each other. Patients who are not too well can lie on beds in the adjoining small rooms, but most of us sit in the chairs, often with family, friends and carers. There is a radio and CD player on a book cabinet which contains some old favourites. The music plays softly in the background. The TV is on at special times, like the Grand Final Parade.

The nurses are like family now. Familiar faces, warm smiles. A hug if you need it, or a shoulder to cry on. They go about their business, appearing with the injection or attaching the intravenous bag of life-saving drugs. There is no fuss. They are diligent, watching each patient to see that all is well. A volunteer helps, handing around drinks, sandwiches and fruit, or just spending time with patients who are by themselves.

I feel safe and protected. It's odd, considering the reason I am here, but I actually look forward to my days here. The patients know each other and exchange stories, but we don't dwell on why we're here. There's no need. We all know that we are either fighting for a cure or fighting to stay alive for as long as possible, living with the diagnosis of advanced breast cancer.

On the day of my last treatment, the needle is injected and the drip is on its way when a lady appears for the first time. She is to start her first chemotherapy treatment. She tentatively sits down in a seat near me. I can see the fear in her eyes. I remember feeling like that five years ago. I could actually taste the fear. She asks if she can be put into one of the rooms away from everyone. It would be a good idea to start out here, the nurse tells her, maybe later she might feel like moving. This does not go down well. She is close to tears. All the other patients are talking, laughing at jokes, reading books, sharing stories. The new patient is given a rundown on her treatment, what to expect and how to manage any possible side effects. She looks as if she is about to flee. The intravenous drip is connected to her. The volunteer offers her a drink and something to eat. The gentleman next to her introduces himself and all the other patients close by follow.

As I leave an hour later, she is not so frightened. She is holding a hot drink, relating her story to the person next to her and actually laughing. She has stayed in the circle. She might come to think of it as a warm, inviting place to visit, as it has been for me.

Carolyn Johnson

Chocolate frogs

Elephants and clogs

*M*y surgeon's desk is crowded. The elephants' trunks are raised high, their bodies carved from smooth grey rock. Beside them stand a pair of clogs, their wooden toes turned upward, painted in vivid yellows and reds. Reaching above them is the metallic spire of the Eiffel Tower. The entire surface of the antique wooden desk is a field of figures in wood, plastic, metal, china and glass of all colours, crowding the phone and prescription pad.

There's Mickey Mouse with his wind-up key, a heavy lead nail from a railway track and a glass crystal suspended within a glass frame. Sunlight from the window is captured in the crystal and released in a rainbow of colours over the sea of souvenirs. I smile at a bottle, a perfect miniature with its Russian label and half-swallow of vodka.

When I first saw these figures they mocked me, shouting about other people's happy times and dreams, far beyond anything possible for my own life. Or so I had thought. My eyes scanned the desktop. Behind the brilliant red London double-decker, I found him. Standing defiantly, wearing his silver helmet and brandishing his silver sword was my contribution, a Swedish Viking. I had bought him from a small shop in a narrow cobbled laneway in Stockholm to bring home for my oncologist's desktop.

Now, I reach over, pick him up and place him in front of them all. He is a fighter.

Careful steps

Nestled in low-slung canvas chairs, Bruce and I relax on the decking with our cold drinks. The cat rubs against my legs and I reach out to stroke his silky black coat, warmed by the sun. In profile, Alonzo is a perfect sphinx, until he opens his mouth, revealing a misshapen jaw and missing teeth.

In a maelstrom of children's tears, cat howling and blood, we gambled on his fate twelve years ago. The cost of surgery was high and his chance of survival slim, but there was no choice. We refused to allow yet more grief to surround our children, who already feared for their mother. The surgery had gone ahead.

All of his steps were carefully and slowly measured. Alonzo spent hours gently resting and sleeping, curled onto a thick bed of soft leaves beneath a sheltering bush. Nursing my own wounds, I had watched him.

Now, the cat steadies his weight on his back legs and stares fixedly upward. In one muscular fluid leap, he reaches the overhanging grapevine and picks his way to the roof. I smile, lean back with a sigh, and bask in the luxury of our good health.

Theme song

I lay on my back on the firm bed, chest bared and decorated with dark lines. A large circular dish was suspended above and bore down centimetres from my upper body. Careful not to move my head, I glanced sideways to see the heavy lead-lined door. The nurse had left. 'Are you all right Carolyn?' I was and they began.

The high-tech machine barely made a sound as the gamma rays began their work. Closing my eyes I concentrated on using the energy of the rays. Watching them shining into my body. Seeing the cancer cells shrivel and die in their heat. Breathing slowly, deeply. Precious calm began to fill my mind and my body relaxed.

Background music filtered through. They were playing John Farnham. I liked some of his slow songs. Yes, I liked this one. *Burn for you.* The words he was singing became clear and I struggled not to laugh out loud.

Burn for you...What am I going to do?

I burn for you...bur-ur-urn for you.

I so love laughing.

I so love being alive.

Going away

A few people with suitcases at their feet stood quietly in the cool hotel foyer, waiting. A mini-bus pulled up and we moved outside. I turned to Bruce. 'I've changed my mind. I'm coming home. I don't want to be away from you all for so long.' He looked at me with such anxious concern that the guilt surfaced again. What pain I was causing us all! Putting his arm around me he said, 'You'll be fine and we'll be fine too. Wish I was coming though, so give me a ring tonight will you?'

The driver lifted my case into the bus and with a broad smile he said, 'You have made such an important decision. You won't regret coming to Ian Gawler's retreat.' I climbed aboard, lay my hot forehead against the cool glass of the window and waved goodbye.

Special friends

*H*ow long has it been now?' she asks.

'Fifteen years since the start of breast cancer and twelve years with secondaries,' I reply. My friend touches my arm. 'It's because you're special,' she says with affection. 'You've done all the right things.'

I know what she is saying and I appreciate the support and caring, but I am uncomfortable. Many wonderful young women I have known have also done all the right things and they haven't survived.

Throughout that day, I think of them. Annette, fiery-headed, funny and competent, was indispensable to her husband and two very young children. She will always be special. There was Bev and Gabrielle and Doris and Lorinda.

I recall the people I have met on this cancer journey and how we moved beyond pleasantries to real life and death issues. Strangers became soulmates so quickly in our support group. Rhonda, funny and gentle, was always searching for the latest information. She was a loving wife and mother to two young children.

I miss my special friends. They all deserved to live. Sometimes I happen to see their families, now without their wives and mothers. My cancer history gave many of them hope – it is possible to live for much longer than expected.

But they have gone. I find it hard to meet the eyes of their husbands and children. Surely, they must look at me and wonder, 'Why isn't my wife alive?' 'Why isn't my mum alive?'

I chat away and so do they, but there's another conversation running beneath my spoken words. I'm so sorry that she didn't make it. I wish I knew what made the difference. I wish your family had been lucky too. I am just so sorry.

'See you,' I say.

And they say, 'Good to see you.'

Everyone benefits

*M*y oncologist reached into his drawer and pulled out half a dozen small boxes held together by an elastic band. 'Well,' he said, 'This is all I've got. The staff have spent the week ringing pharmacies and hospitals, all over the place, in every state. This is it.' He looked tired and almost defeated.

I was doing well on my current medication, but it wouldn't always work this well. And the next drug for me, Halotestin, was the one he was holding. He had even investigated importing the drug directly from the American manufacturer, but the cost would be huge.

'So, it isn't going out of production then?' I was puzzled.

He told me that since the drug was no longer on the free list, as part of the Pharmaceutical Benefits Scheme, the sales had dropped so the drug company had withdrawn it from sale here.

I leaned forward in my chair. 'But what about the women already on it?'

He shrugged helplessly. 'I'm getting really good results with this, so I'm not sure what I'll do.' He raised his hands in frustration. 'I've emailed the Health Minister every day this week, as a matter of urgency, and haven't had a reply.'

Our PBS is admired all over the world for its success in delivering medicines at affordable prices to everyone who needs them. What is happening here? I left his office anxious and determined to find out more.

Over the next few days the media covered the situation. Some members of the PBS Board resigned in protest, concerned about possible pharmaceutical company and political pressures influencing decisions of the board. Feeling powerless and angry, I sent this letter to *The Age* newspaper:

Dear Sir,

On Friday I visited my oncologist. He had some good news and some bad news. First the good news.

The next drug recommended in my treatment (Halotestin) is successfully extending the lives of many women with advanced breast cancer.

Now for the bad news. This drug is no longer available in Australia, having been withdrawn by its manufacturer, Upjohn-Pharmacia.

The Minister for Health doesn't have a problem with this, having failed to respond to concerns raised over the last year when the drug was taken off the free list and fears for its availability were first realised.

It appears that the priorities for access to drugs now depend, not on their intrinsic value as medication, but on their ability to make profits for company management and shareholders. It's a sorry state of affairs when profits are placed before health.

The latest Government revamping of the highly respected Australian Benefits Advisory Committee gives little hope of improving the situation.

Three months later, back in the surgery, I asked the oncologist about Halotestin. 'Not a problem,' he said with a pleased smile. 'I went higher up, politically, and I have access to the drug. But I really shouldn't have to spend my time playing politics!'

We shouldn't have to fight to protect the best pharmaceutical system in the world, or what is left of it, but maybe we all have to become politically savvy.

The tomato grower

I moved slowly down the footpath, outside once again. The smell of sweet spring air came as a surprise. The pain from my recent operation was a background ache; my strength was slowly returning.

I felt raw; the turmoil of the last few weeks had stripped me of so much. I had lost the innocence of good health and the plans for a future based on the casual assumption that there would BE a future. I mourned the loss of my old familiar role as a wife, mother, daughter, friend, teacher and future grandparent. Everything was changing. I mourned for the person I would never be. My brain felt bruised from dealing with pain and fear. I needed a walk.

My neighbour lifted his head from where he had been pulling weeds. Himid was originally from the old Yugoslavia, and forty years in Australia and an Australian family haven't robbed him of his accent.

'Hallo,' he said with a smile and a studied look. 'How are you?' His was more than caring concern. He had been dealing with stomach cancer, in some form or other, for twenty years. His method of staying well was very simple.

'I fill up my wheelbarrow with bricks and in the middle of the night when I can't sleep…the pain can get bad, you know…I get up and run around the outside of my house, pushing that barrow. Now I am not too bad.'

Himid leases a farm where he grows tomatoes that he sells locally. His days are long and physically demanding. Twice weekly during the season he loads his truck with crates of tomatoes and drives two hours to Melbourne's Queen Vic market. Hard work is his answer and he certainly lives it out. No one dares criticise his chain smoking!

'Well Himid,' I reply, 'I'm feeling a bit better, I think largely because the shock is beginning to wear off.' Himid's face turned red and he waved his hands about furiously.

'SHOCK!' he yelled. 'You tell me about SHOCK. When

those bloody doctors tell me I have three months to live, it takes me TWO YEARS to get over that shock.' His fury still grips him as I laugh helplessly.

He looks at me saying, 'What? What?'

Thank you Himid, for a much-needed belly laugh and a new perspective when I really needed one. How good it is to meet people who defy the odds!

Undone

The twins play netball.
Their legs and arms are long and thin.
Too young and vulnerable.
I won't be here to protect them.
And I am undone.

The children enter my hospital room,
Faltering as they see bottles and tubes.
Wide-eyed and pale
They move close to their father
And I am undone.

I return to hospital
Sandbagged by infection.
Strained and hesitant, my son asks
'Mum, are you dying?'
And I am undone.

After a check-up, my son says
'I knew you'd do well.'
But I saw his first glance
Fearful and anxious
And I am undone.

My husband is positive.
But I know his sleepless nights.
His face reflects worry and fear.
What pain I am causing!
And I am undone.

My parents shift closer.
They watch over me,
The old agony of losing a son
Awakened in their eyes.

174

And I am undone.

And now –
I drink in the faces of my adult children.
I float in their laughter.
I am filled with gratitude and love
And I am undone.

Biographies

These biographies were written by the contributors during the course of the writing project. Since that time, some of the contributors have died.

Trish Armstrong

I was born in Melbourne. I lived for fifteen years in country Victoria and NSW, returning to Melbourne fourteen years ago. I have a daughter who has returned from overseas living with me, and a son in the army who lives in Townsville. I had a mastectomy in 1998 followed by chemotherapy. In 2002 I was diagnosed with metastatic cancer in the liver, lung and bones, followed by a further diagnosis in the brain – almost four years to the day from my first diagnosis of breast cancer. I left work and continued to have treatment, concentrating on the healing process.

Lyn Clarke

I was first diagnosed with breast cancer in November 2002. At the time I was working, putting far too much energy into the business my wonderful bloke and I had recently purchased from our long-term partners. There was no turning back with the bank loan looming and the business booming.

The catalyst for my diagnosis was a really bad back and my 'deal with it later' secret, a lump in my breast. My treatment was rapid radiotherapy on my spine, then chemo, followed by a mastectomy, more chemo and more radiotherapy. I went on Femara, heaving a sigh of relief as it took effect.

I live in Mackay, North Queensland. I have six children who light my life and a pretty okay husband who has amassed lots of brownie points. I was first published in the *Beezer* in 1967, and have written as a hobby for years. I found the writing project an enriching and enlightening part of my blessed life.

Gayle Creed

I was first diagnosed in 1998 at thirty-nine after I found a lump and went to my local GP. My tests were positive, so I went to see a specialist, then I had surgery. I had a lumpectomy followed two weeks later by a modified radical mastectomy. I had twenty-eight doses of radiation followed by Tamoxifen, a treatment that was reduced to three months due to side effects. For the next two-and-a-half years I went for regular check-ups, followed various doctors' orders and tried to get on with life.

During this time though, something didn't feel quite right. None of the check-ups or tests showed anything out of the ordinary until February 2001. CT scans followed and the diagnosis was confirmed. The cancer had spread to my bones.

At that point my family and I fell apart. Breast Cancer Network Australia was a lifeline. I heard about it through our franchisor, Bakers Delight. I have taken radical steps and drastic measures since the metastatic diagnosis, and so has my family.

I am planning to do everything I can and enjoy as much time as I can: 'Life's too short, eat dessert first!'

Mary Dewhurst

At fifty-four I was living in Glenbrook, a wonderful community-spirited hamlet in the Blue Mountains with my husband and my four-legged best mate Zeus (well, three-legged, as a result of an altercation with an XPT). My daughter was studying at the University of New England, Armidale, my grandson was eight and my twin granddaughters were two. I had a lumpectomy for a benign breast lump in 1992, but in 1997 I was diagnosed with breast cancer in the same breast. I had another lumpectomy, radiotherapy and my ovaries were removed. I got the 'all clear', but then, in 2002, I was told I had metastatic cancer in my liver and bones.

My journey has been awful and wonderful. The reality of cancer is heart-wrenching and painful. Death is more real. Priorities are quickly reshuffled. Time spent with family and friends is appreciated on a deeper level. Discovering the 'no' word was empowering. It's no longer crucial to mop the kitchen floor every day and I am acting on my 'must do' list. At home I can step outside, look at the forest of giant Turpentine trees swaying gracefully, listen to the birds singing and think myself lucky.

Leona Furstenburg

I was thirty-seven and married to the man of my dreams, Roy. We were living in Canberra and had a golden retriever pup, Max. I was diagnosed with breast cancer in February 2000. I was treated with a lumpectomy with axillary clearance, followed by high-dose chemotherapy with stem cell support, and then six weeks of radiotherapy. Less than three years later, the cancer returned in the lymph system in my neck. I was treated with four different regimes of chemotherapy and each time a new tumour appeared. Subsequently I had radiotherapy.

I am involved with my local ACT breast cancer support group, Bosom Buddies. The friends I have met there give me constant support and friendship. Life is challenging, but Roy and I continue to fight with the strength and love we share, and hope that one day things will get better. We live life to the full, enjoying our many shared interests and taking nothing for granted.

Annie Hall

I live in Mount Riverview in the Blue Mountains. I was diagnosed with breast cancer in 1996 at thirty-seven. A lumpectomy and radiation followed. A rethink of values came about and in 1999, one of my dreams was fulfilled when my husband, twelve-year-old daughter and I flew to South America, and from there embarked on an expedition to Antarctica.

In 2003, at forty-three, I was diagnosed with advanced breast cancer in the liver and bones. I started on hormone treatment and am well, with the disease fairly stable.

I love my husband, daughter, shih-tzu Lorelai, reading, travel, music, patchwork, theatre, walking and spending precious time with family and friends. My belief is that each day is a gift. Advanced breast cancer is a journey of highs and lows, great joys and great sorrows. There has been much learning and stumbling, but I have continued to pick myself up, even when it's almost too difficult. There are days of great pride and happiness at what I am able to achieve, and also days of frustration when time seems to slip through my fingers. I try to live in the moment, which, when you think about it, is all anyone really has.

Lee-anne Hazeldene

I am forty, divorced, and have three children aged fifteen, thirteen and eight. I live in Benalla, in north-east Victoria.

In December 1997 I was diagnosed with breast cancer. I had a lumpectomy and a full nodal clearance on the left side. Then I had a second operation, a mastectomy, on the same breast. In 1998 I underwent six months of chemotherapy, leaving me with a rocky marriage. In 1999 I divorced my husband and only gained fifty per cent custody of my children. In June 2000 I was diagnosed with a tumour in my head which was surgically removed. Radiotherapy caused me to lose all the hair on my head. In August 2002, another tumour was found in my spinal column. Surgery and radiotherapy followed. During 2003, I suffered pain in my back, then in October they found a spot on my bones.

My journey has been very stressful; waiting to hear about the next course of treatment and this latest diagnosis. I am very keen to tell my story so other women in similar circumstances may be able to draw strength from my writing. I enjoy each day, being as happy and involved in life as I can be!

Carolyn Johnson

I am fifty-two, live in Bendigo, am wife to Bruce, and mother to two boys aged thirty and twenty-nine and twin girls aged twenty-four. Fifteen years ago, while teaching and studying, I developed breast cancer. Three years later it was in my breastbone and neck and arm lymph glands. Radiotherapy, surgery and hormone treatment were used through the following years. I taught until another setback six years ago. I am stable on hormone treatment.

Life has had its highs in this challenging time, including living in Sweden, riding in a hot air balloon, snorkelling, doing tapestry, Tai Chi, meditation, church life, daily walks and talks, riding a bike again and having golf lessons. By far, the thing I most cherish is precious family get-togethers. I have worked with a boy with autism for the last eight years and my family has provided respite care for children with disabilities. I have contributed towards establishing the Otis Units in Bendigo, at which people with a breast cancer history are invited to spend time out, free of charge.

Mary McGregor

One hour after a rigorous basketball game, I was wondering why my right breast was sore. Hysterics set in when I felt the hard, swollen breast. My life changed. Within a week I was undergoing tests for breast cancer. A rare form – inflammatory breast cancer – was diagnosed and within ten days I began a long journey of chemotherapy, mastectomy and radiotherapy. It was hard to believe that this had happened to me, a fit, full-of-life, fifty-five-year-old primary school principal. Life had been crammed with travelling adventures, sporting achievements and workplace challenges.

Once over the initial shock I was determined to lead my life as normally as possible. I continued to pursue my professional role, with my colleagues and school community members providing wonderful support. I also continued to be physically active, and participated in the World Masters Games in Melbourne in the week between chemotherapy and mastectomy. Without immediate family, my relationships with close friends became more important and intensive. My extended friendship networks are kept up-to-date through regular emailed journal articles.

My resilience continued throughout my treatment. Since the end of treatment, life is different. I am linked to the fragility of life itself and have a greater appreciation of human nature. I look forward to many healthy years.

Veronica Macaulay-Cross

I was a forty-year-old secondary teacher when I found a lump and was diagnosed with breast cancer in 1996. At the time, my daughter was ten. The treatment was a mastectomy and tram flap reconstruction, followed by chemotherapy. In May 1997, I found a localised recurrence which required surgery and radiotherapy. Unfortunately, in mid-1999, a cough and sore hip led to the diagnosis of metastatic breast cancer in my bones (spine) and lungs. Second line chemotherapy cleared the lungs and shrank the cancer in the bones. Four years on, my breast cancer continues to respond to treatment. Firstly, anti-oestrogen medication and bisphosphonate treatment, then Xeloda chemotherapy.

I generally enjoy a good quality of life. My husband and

parents are extremely supportive. I am passionate about equity and accessibility of treatment and support for women with breast cancer. Although 'state of the art' drugs, treatment and support are costly, I argue that the contribution women make to our society more than compensates. Quality of life must be paramount in the management of treatments. I am an active consumer representative and am working in Queensland to form cooperative links with other breast cancer agencies. I enjoy travel, the beach and spending time with family and friends.

Pat Mathew

At fifty-five, I have been married to Peter for thirty-six years. We have three sons, one daughter and five grandchildren. I am the eldest of ten children. Just before our mother died, she summoned the family to her side and announced that I was now to be the matriarch. For a while this responsibility weighed heavily on my shoulders, and I felt that I should be dressing the part in a long skirt and headscarf. Now though, informality and comfort best describe my sartorial style, and I usually wear shorts or comfortable trousers.

I am happiest when surrounded by family and friends, in the kitchen or in the garden. A pantry full of bottled fruit, jams and sauces and a freezer full of summer vegetables gives me a lot of satisfaction. Peter and I lived on a hobby farm while our children were growing up, and are now semi-retired in Devonport. We have enjoyed several long caravanning holidays on mainland Australia, and particularly enjoy Tasmania's national parks and coastal reserves. I was diagnosed with breast cancer in 1996, and have undergone surgery, two courses of radiotherapy and three different lots of chemotherapy.

Jenny Morrison

I had just completed a wonderful two-kilometre swim and cycled home when I noticed something 'different' near my collarbone. It signalled the beginning of ongoing changes in my life. I was forty-seven, fit and healthy and loved outdoor activities.

I had a lumpectomy in February 1997 and was placed on Tamoxifen. The shock of having breast cancer lasted a long while, only to be overtaken some three-and-a-half years later when the cancer progressed to my femur and thoracic spine. Fortunately, a close friend moved in to support me through the roller-coaster ride that has come to characterise my life. Friends have become even more important. My taste in books has expanded since retiring from a busy professional life.

My disease has progressed to other bones, and to my liver and lung. The treatment has become more aggressive. I have moved through several forms of chemotherapy. Unfortunately, I have not been able to swim or walk regularly since being hospitalised for three weeks, which is frustrating. Having always been a planner, I have learned to live one day at a time.

I have learnt to knit and this gives me a sense of accomplishment. I ache to swim regularly, and I enjoy the outdoors when I can.

Jenny Muller

I was diagnosed with breast cancer in August 1996 at forty-four. Though it's been a demanding time, there have been plenty of blessings. My husband John, my parents and my family have been a wonderful support. Through this time my two lovely stepsons, aged twenty-three and twenty-eight, have had a difficult time – their mother died of breast cancer in 2001.

In 1996 I had chemotherapy then a mastectomy. In 1997 I had chemo and a stem cell transplant, then chest wall radiotherapy and some time on Tamoxifen. In 1997 I attended the Gawler ten-day program. With an 'all clear' at the end of 1997, I had a go at a few hours of work per week. Unfortunately, around autumn 1998 I started to get hip pain, a funny walk, then rib pain. The scans showed lots of spots. I started on Pamidronate and changed from Tamoxifen to Letrozole. After trying all the then-available anti-inflammatory painkillers, I was prescribed slow release morphine. I continued to get sicker with pain on movement, limb swelling and left arm lymphoedema. In mid-1999 I had an inpatient stay at a rehabilitation hospital to check for arthritis and to have physio and hydrotherapy. Now I can walk to the pool and swim! In 2000 I changed from Letrozole to Provera, and took Capecitabine (Xeloda) for a few months. I stopped Provera in December and in February 2001 started Herceptin. In March I stopped the morphine, in April I stopped the Celebrex, and felt great!

Julie Pallot

I live in Melbourne with my three daughters. I was first diagnosed with breast cancer in June 1993, the day after my fortieth birthday. I had a lumpectomy, gland clearance and six weeks of radiation. Unfortunately, in May 1995 it was found that cancer had spread to the bones. I underwent more radiation treatment and my ovaries were radiated. Over the following few years, I had most of the hormone treatments available to control outbreaks in my lungs, liver, lymphatic system and bones. In 1998, I was diagnosed with a large tumour in my femur (thigh bone) and underwent radical surgery to have the femur removed, which included a hip replacement. In 2001, I needed to have chemotherapy for the first time. I participated in a trial of Capecitabine (Xeloda), a daily tablet form of chemotherapy, which was successful. I had another round of Xeloda in 2003 with good results. I turned fifty and therefore am in my second decade of the disease.

I am an active member of Breast Cancer Network Australia and am on BCNA's Advanced Breast Cancer Working Party. In 2003 I undertook BCNA's Advocacy and Science Training and am committed to improving the quality of services for, and understanding of, advanced breast cancer.

My interests are gardening, sewing and spending time with family and friends.

Anne Pennington

I was originally diagnosed with breast cancer in October 1999 at forty-seven. With tumours in both breasts, I underwent a bi-lateral mastectomy followed by a six-month course of chemotherapy. I was first diagnosed with metastatic spread to the bones in August 2001. Since then the cancer has spread to lymph nodes in my neck, my bone marrow and my liver. I take Letrazole, and have monthly Zometa.

However, after five chemotherapy treatments, I was informed that there were no further treatments that would achieve the desired results without significant side effects. My treatment has changed to be palliative in nature, where symptoms are treated to achieve maximum quality of life for as long as possible.

I am a member of both Breast Cancer Network Australia and Breast Cancer Action Group. I undertook BCNA's Advocacy and

Science Training in 2001. I have represented consumers on a number of committees, including being a member of BCNA's Advanced Breast Cancer Working Party.

I live in Benalla in north-east Victoria, supported by a caring husband, family, and a large circle of friends.

Judy Shepherdson

In 1993 with my youngest starting school, after ten years of hard mothering and having had four children under five, I planned to reclaim my life. I was going to return to study, wanting to learn about horticulture. Gardening was my passion. I wanted to learn to swim and play golf. April Fool's Day brought a diagnosis of breast cancer. Surgery, chemotherapy and radiotherapy meant a year of grief and lost dreams. In December 1994 came re-diagnosis and more surgery. In 1995 I had radiotherapy. Mid-year I had my ovaries ablated with radiotherapy, causing instant menopause. In 1996 I attempted to pick up the threads of my life. In 1997 and 1998 I was coming to terms with living under a cloud of uncertainty. In 1999, fulfilling a dream, I moved to the country and opened a shop, 'Isabella Rose – Something Old, Something New.' Life was carefree for three years. In 2002, my cancer returned. I had both breasts removed and received the devastating news of spread to my right lung. Isabella Rose closed. In 2003, my marriage of twenty-seven years ended.

Breast cancer has brought many wonderful people into my life. I am passionate about the issues for rural/remote women and raising awareness of their difficulties. A friend told me, 'Only the good die young, and you will live forever because you do bad so well!' I treasure my friendships. They sustain and nourish my soul. I live life to capacity, savouring every precious moment.

Monique Skarke

I have worked in a variety of professions, attained tertiary and post-graduate qualifications, lived alone and as a de-facto partner, travelled to far away places, and enjoyed many of life's treats.

At thirty-four, I gave birth to my son, Gabriel, whose father Carlo has been my partner for over five-and-a-half years. We are a two-car, two-cat, single income family who don't get to spend enough time together.

In October 2001, I was diagnosed with breast cancer and underwent a lumpectomy, six months of chemotherapy and radiotherapy. Then began the long, anxious wait to see if the treatment had worked. In November 2002, I received the all clear. However, in August 2003 I stepped onto the cancer merry-go-round again when I was diagnosed with a recurrence of the cancer in my lungs. Chemotherapy was advocated, and a lifetime of antibody therapy.

I have managed to maintain a positive outlook because I have realised that many of life's worst moments bring with them some of life's most valuable lessons! I have met wonderful people since my breast cancer diagnosis.

I have vowed to take it one week at a time, while also trying to enjoy what each new day has to offer. My greatest challenge is trying to balance my own needs with the requirements of being the mother of a toddler.

Bronwyn Taylor

My friends know never to call before breakfast. When I finally get up, I fill in each moment of the day, often until past midnight. When I confided to a friend that the chemo had slowed me down a little, the friend looked thrilled and said I would now be on a par with the rest of civilisation.

I had just finished breast-feeding Benjamin when I noticed a lump that had not gone away. A week later I was in the botanical gardens telling my parents the bad news while baby Benjamin toddled round the bandstand.

Ten operations later, I have managed to keep up my playgroup for children with special needs, plus some kindergarten teaching, which is my great love. I have also taken on a variety of community positions and voluntary work, which earned me the Moira Shire Citizen of the Year award in 2001. I have also been nominated for the Rural Women Roll of Honour. I love to sew, garden (especially with bulbs and propagating cuttings), take photos, read historical novels, write, and wander around the wetland and bushland my family has helped create at the end of the street.

I am ably supported by myriad friends, my parents, my five young nephews and their parents. I am especially proud of my wonderful husband, three noisy and enthusiastic children, and four chooks.

Maria Waters

I was born in Perth in 1954, and had a traditional Italian upbringing. I shared my childhood with an elder brother, younger sister and a multitude of cousins. Educated at a private college, I left school at fifteen and worked in an office where I met my husband Alan. We married in 1980, our first son was born in 1983, and our second son eighteen months later. I have dabbled in pottery and china painting, and have played tennis and squash. Although I'm not throwing clay any longer, I enjoy browsing through art and craft stores. I enjoy completing crosswords, working needlework, going to the football and most of all, baking while my favourite Elvis CD is playing. The diagnosis of breast cancer in 1989 was a shock. To be told of advanced disease three years later was devastating. This was the start of a long and challenging battle. I continue to strive towards the future, living with advanced breast cancer, in a stable condition.

Lesley Wilder

I am forty-eight, live in Brisbane, am wife to Clive and mother to a large extended family. Diagnosed with invasive ductile carcinoma in my left breast in 1992, I underwent a lumpectomy, excision of lymph nodes, chemotherapy and radiotherapy. For eight years I remained well, though busy with my family and full-time work as a conveyancer in a suburban law firm. I am an avid crocheter, and when I was diagnosed with extensive secondaries to my liver, lungs and bones in 2000, I set myself the task of making baby things for the grandchildren I feared I would not live to see. Following chemotherapy in 2001, the tumours in my liver and lungs were gone, and those in my bones were stable. Progression in 2002 was once again stabilised by treatment. I am receiving chemotherapy for progression in my liver. Having prepared for my imminent demise, I have since come to terms with living, and am revelling in it.

For more information

Some established services and information providers for women with advanced breast cancer and organisations, books and websites about advanced breast cancer are listed here. This list is not comprehensive. Details were correct at the time of printing.

Breast Cancer Network Australia
1800 500 258
www.bcna.org.au
beacon@bcna.org.au
293 Camberwell Road, Camberwell Vic 3124

Breast Cancer Network Australia publishes *The Inside Story* about secondary breast cancer (a quarterly supplement to its *Beacon* magazine) and the booklet *Messages of Hope and Inspiration from Women Living with Advanced Breast Cancer* and lists resources and support groups on its website about secondary breast cancer.

National Breast Cancer Centre
1800 624 973
www.nbcc.org.au
directorate@nbcc.org.au
92 Parramatta Road, Camperdown NSW 2050

Publications include *A Guide for Women with Metastatic Breast Cancer, Clinical Practice Guidelines for the Management of Advanced Breast Cancer,* and *Clinical Practice Guidelines for the Psychosocial Care of Adults with Cancer.*

BreaCan
1300 781 500
breacan@breacan.org.au
www.whv.org.au/breacan
Ground floor, Queen Victoria Women's Centre
210 Lonsdale Street, Melbourne Vic 3000

BreaCan offers information sessions and an eight-week program for Victorian women living with advanced breast cancer, as well as a free, confidential information, support and referral service.

Choices for Women with Advanced Breast Cancer
1800 227 271 or (07) 3232 7064
choices@wesley.com.au
choices.wesley.com.au

A Queensland support network for women diagnosed with secondary breast cancer based in Brisbane and conducted by The Wesley Hospital Kim Walters Choices Program.

Group for Women with Advanced Breast Cancer, Queensland
(07) 3217 2998
www.advancedbreastcancergroup.org
wps2@bigpond.net.au

Rural and regional women in Queensland can join the Brisbane-based meetings by teleconference. The moderated forums and online support on the group's website are open to all Australians affected by secondary breast cancer.

Living Well forums
13 11 20 Cancer Helpline
www.cancervic.org.au
enquiries@cancervic.org.au

One-day forums for people with advanced cancer, their families and friends run by The Cancer Council Victoria.

Advanced Breast Cancer: A Guide to Living with Metastatic Disease
2nd edition, 1998, by Musa Mayer, published by O'Reilly and Associates

Dr Susan Love's Breast Book
4th edition, 2005, by Dr Susan M Love with Karen Lindsey, published by Da Capo Press

Contains useful information about secondary breast cancer.

Aussie Breast Cancer Forum
www.bcaus.org.au

An online forum with an advanced breast cancer section.

BCMets.org – Metastatic Breast Cancer Information and Support
www.bcmets.org

A US website and forum for secondary breast cancer.

Cancerbackup: Secondary Breast Cancer Information Centre
www.cancerbackup.org.uk/Cancertype/Breastsecondary

A UK website on secondary breast cancer that includes information about secondary sites and treatment options.

Index by title